# WHAT COMES AFTER

# CANCER

A memoir for patients, family, and friends
dealing with critical illness

**Patricia Rodi**

*WHAT COMES AFTER CANCER* is a work of non-fiction.

Editor:  Claire Holden Rothman
Cover Photo:  N'Focus By Dory
Author Photo:  William Brock
Makeup Artist:  Antoinette Orofino
Cover Design:  Patricia Rodi

**ISBN** 978-1-7778189-0-6 (Paperback, Oxford English)
**ISBN** 978-1-7778189-1-3 (Paperback, US Edition)

## Praise for *WHAT COMES AFTER CANCER*

"This riveting memoir tells the story of a Montreal woman's experience after being diagnosed... Walking us through the lengthy, challenging process of the cure, the book offers an insider's view of a life-threatening disease and survival."

Award-winning writer **Claire Holden Rothman**

"A moving story of a cancer survivor, written from the heart."

Award-winning writer **Joan Hall Hovey**

## PLEDGE:

The HOPE & COPE WELLNESS CENTRE, a volunteer-based cancer foundation helping families since 1981, will benefit from the profits of this book.

*For my one and only... Isabella. There are no words to define it and no actions to prove it... only the profound love I feel when you look at me.*

# TABLE OF CONTENTS

# Chapter 1

# Flying to Freedom

*We are born alone. We die alone.*

L ate summer, 2017, we arrive in Cuba in the middle of the night, hungry and tired out by the travel from airport to airport and a long bus ride to our resort. When we check in, the receptionist tells us there is a 24-hour restaurant on the property, so we're soon eating grilled chicken burgers and fries before turning in. I take note of the location. I have a feeling I'll be using it.

These all-inclusives are my favourite vacations. I have to eat often, so it is a relief knowing there is always an open kitchen. It's been a long road to recovery, and I am finally spending time with my family without having to exhaust my energy cooking, doing chores, or being sick. I am looking forward to being with my 14-year-old daughter, Isabella, to help her forget the harder days of the past.

The next morning, as we step outside of our second floor, orange-themed resort room, Isabella looks for the baby iguana she found lingering around the light of our hallway door. Though she thinks it's the cutest thing, and looks forward to catching a glimpse every day, she is secretly afraid of it. We follow it until it disappears into the brush.

We head toward the stairs in the center of the two-story building. The concrete roof protects only the hallways, but the thriving vegetation that separates the guest room hallways loves the rainfall. The four corners of the building on the top floor offer balcony views and the first floor open exits. At the bottom of the stairs a wide, doorless opening leads us to the reception area and most of the restaurants, including the breakfast buffet. The walk is pleasant, with lush green trees and colourful flowers, not to mention larger iguanas camouflaged in the greenery or in plain sight on the walkways. They always seem to be frozen in time with their still, long bodies and blank stare. The restaurant is about 200 steps away, and we pass through the reception area where Isabella hooks up to Wi-Fi to check in with her friends back home in Montreal.

"Come on, Honey, I'm hungry."

"I had trouble connecting…this Wi-Fi is so slow. I'm almost done sending my streaks." She continues swiping and typing. "One more second."

The omelet chef will soon get to know us well, knowing our order even before we ask for it. He's a popular guy at this resort, and I wonder how his arm isn't sore from scrambling each egg order individually. I'm able to finish about half of my veggie and onion omelet, five or six small-cubed roasted potatoes, half a slice of buttered country-style bread, and some of the luscious mango most guests anxiously awaited after each meal. I fold a couple of croissants, pastry, and a banana in napkins to take to the beach. Then we head back to the room to freshen up. I discretely catch my breath from climbing the 20 or so steps at the center of the building, my legs aching.

"Let's hurry, guys, or I'll be hungry again." I lie down on the unmade bed to digest breakfast until my husband, Mariano, and Isabella are ready.

Minutes later, we're walking toward the beach path. Another 200 steps or so... I'm glad our room is located centrally between the beach and the dining room.

"Oh, look, we can try lunch at this buffet today." I am excited at the venue so close to the beach. Staff is already setting the tables.

"We just finished breakfast, Patricia," says Mariano, raising an eyebrow.

"I can come here to eat when it opens. You and Isabella can come later, and I'll join you so I can eat again."

We cross the beach with towels from the towel bar, and I look for a quiet spot. It's getting late and places are scarce. Mariano walks quickly to the far end of the beach-chair-and-umbrella-rows and sets us up. When I finally catch up, out of breath from the heat and the walk, I drop my bag and take in the view.

The lounging chairs are extremely heavy for me to drag. "Can I have my chair in the sun, please?" I feel terrible having to rely on my family to do things for me.

"Me too," Isabella adds.

Cuba's beaches are divine and the sea a warm bath, calm and soothing. The water is so clear you can see the white sand below, sifting over your feet. It's quite peaceful by the shore without the surf forcing you to raise your voice when hanging around the edge of the water. The salt water splashing on my lips may be the only unpleasant thing about this vacation. The trees are lush and green, including the native Royal Palm, which are making a slapping sound as winds move the leaves back and forth. On the beach, some palm trees slant toward the sea, creating a large patch of shade in the late afternoon. The beach umbrella tops are stitched together with ancient, shredded palm branches. Some have been ripped out by strong winds. Those umbrellas are left for late-comers.

I notice scattered flower bushes along the resort paths. One of them is Cuba's National flower. The gardeners we passed each morning told us it is a White Ginger flower or La Mariposa – because its shape resembles a butterfly. It gives off the sweet jasmine scent that pervades the resort grounds. Another one of my favourite flowers was the Heliconia, because they look like what we know as birds of paradise. For me, these flowers represent strength and persistence. Shades of reds and oranges create year-round gardens here, a welcome contrast to the sleet and ice-covered branches back home.

The people that take care of us are friendly, despite the poverty that we know is the norm outside the manicured gardens of this resort. We caught glimpses of the real Cuba on the drive from the airport. We are complicit with this poverty, just by staying here. But I tell myself that the country of Cuba relies on tourism to survive. I hope that by spending hard earned Canadian dollars here, my little family is doing more good than harm to the amazing people who tend to us and to our needs each day of this vacation.

Facing the least-populated corner of the beach, I remove my beach wrap discretely to reveal my scrawny, pale body in a bikini. I am 48 years of age and am currently weighing in at 108 pounds, much less than a healthy woman of my height ought to weigh. Not so long ago I felt like I was 88 years of age. Today, things feel better, but I am still timid about my scars and rake-thin appearance. I stash the wrap in my bag and sit on the lounging chair, leaning forward and resting my hands on my lap, letting my arms conceal the little rolls on my belly. I ask my daughter if she wants to come with me into the water, and she nods.

We walk quickly over the hot sand, and immerse our scorched feet in the tropical seawater. I am amazed to

# Chapter 2

# The Diagnosis

*Before I was diagnosed with cancer, I really didn't know myself at all.*

In March of 2004, I came down with a sore throat. I had a bad cold, but my throat was so irritated that it brought on vomiting. What I experienced next initiated a chain of events that upended my life.

We've all felt that trickling tickle in the throat – the one you can't ever entirely clear by coughing or drinking water. You suck on medicated candy to numb it, and hot liquids only help for a few minutes. Clearing your throat repeatedly just aggravates it. There are times the pain extends into the ear. You try to reach deep inside with your pinky, to scratch what feels like an insect eating away at your eardrum.

Then the cough started. I ran to the washroom gagging, and just made it. When I opened my eyes and looked in the toilet, red splotches dotted the water.

I cleaned up, brushed my teeth, and returned to the bedroom, where Mariano was lying in bed. "I just vomited blood." The cold or virus I had been tending to all week seemed trivial.

"You probably just burst a vessel."

"It was bright red… Something doesn't feel right." I thought for a moment. "I'll call Info-Santé." The nurses on the hotline, available 24 hours a day, can assess a medical situation and make recommendations.

My call went right through. A nurse asked me about pain and stools. She also asked if I'd had any strange symptoms recently. The only unusual moment I could remember was that about three weeks earlier I had felt pain between my breasts – where the esophagus meets the stomach – after eating. I don't remember what I was eating, but the pain was excruciating. It felt as though my food couldn't pass into the stomach. I had not omitted to chew or taken too much at once – I'm not one to gulp down my food. Once the pain subsided, I didn't think much more about it. And there was one more strange thing. "I did notice that yesterday or this morning, I can't remember exactly when… my stools were so dark they looked purple."

"Black," she corrected. "Digested blood. I believe you may be hemorrhaging. You should go to the Emergency Room."

"Really?" The thought of leaving our comfortable bed to go sit in a hospital waiting room for endless hours felt grueling.

I told my husband what the nurse had said and he propped himself up on one elbow. "I don't think it's urgent enough to go to the hospital during the night." He tried to convince the both of us, as he lay in bed. "Tomorrow."

He had said the same thing when I went into labour about a year and a half earlier, which also took place around the same hour – right after he got into bed for the night.

Mariano soon agreed to go to the hospital with me. I am trying to remember who I called to come and look after Isabella, but it's a blank. Chemo brain truly exists. I think it was my mother. I don't think I would have phoned my sisters so late at night since they worked the next day.

The half-empty waiting room was filled with black chairs, attached by their feet to the floor, no colour on the walls to lighten the mood, and very little action in calling patients to see the doctor – if there even was one at that ungodly hour. It was tough to stay awake, but I could not doze off on those germ-ridden chairs. Mariano bowed his head and slept.

It was such a long night, but I was determined to get answers. We were frustrated by the time three a.m. came around, but stayed until I was called at seven fifteen that morning.

The doctor requested blood work, and results showed I was anemic. "I have Thalassaemia Minor," I told her, since I knew the two conditions looked similar in test results.

My family doctor had recently explained to me that Thalassaemia, an inherited blood disorder that can result in abnormal or insufficient hemoglobin in the blood, shows as anemia. By checking ferritin reserves, the two conditions can be differentiated. I wonder if knowing that I was also anemic would have made any difference in the timing of my diagnosis. As it turned out, my hemoglobin deficiency was more than likely related to blood loss through my stools.

Since no results other than a low blood count caused concern that day, I was sent home. Would it have made much difference waiting until the next day to go to the hospital? Would I have gone on my own or tried to see my family doctor following the spitting of blood or new stool colour? No other symptoms occurred for quite some time, so surely I would have done what most people do... forgotten about it.

The emergency doctor handled my case with great care. She never gave up on trying to identify the source of the blood – even after I left the local hospital that day. For two months, until the end of May, I alternated between visits with her and medical tests. I was indifferent about the investigation, and made no connection with having spit blood or the stomach pain. But the preparation of some of those tests she scheduled was dreadful.

My insides have been subject to magnetic resonance imaging, ultrasound, barium meal testing, and a colonoscopy. Nothing was discovered as the cause of the blood or pain. The doctor did explain that, since all the other organs were clean, the problem lay somewhere between the mouth and the bowel.

Each time I'm at the ocean and my lips taste the saltwater, I remember the bowel-cleanser I had to drink prior to invasive interventions like the colonoscopy. Just a few drops on my lips make me gag. Forcing the entire sodium phosphate solution down was not easy. Even the chalky barium meal preparation tasted better.

Although the emergency physician confirmed that my colonoscopy was clear, she had concerns about the upper torso. The organs were all clean, but she would send me to a gastroenterologist.

The wait time for meeting that specialist was about two and a half months. When I finally met him, I didn't like him. He seemed angry that I wasn't thrilled he would stick a tube down my throat and into my stomach - while awake - to see what was wrong.

The frightened look on my face during our initial consultation on August 17 surely said it all. The doctor was silent as he pulled out a picture from his desk drawer and handed it to me. Obviously, I wasn't the only one who needed convincing of this helpful procedure. He held a piece of rubber tubing in the other hand. "This tube has a camera attached to the end of it. It is the *only* way to see this." He pointed to the bloody esophagus.

I turned my head away for a second. It was just a picture of the inside of an esophagus, but it made me cringe. It's not easy to picture what goes on inside, especially when something has gone wrong.

How much longer could I put off the inevitable? By this time, the pain from swallowing was frequent, so the gastroenterologist scheduled a test soon after, but got rescheduled twice. It was eventually done on September 8.

The gastroscopy was horrific. Not as traumatizing as the tube, the anesthetic spray in my throat was gagworthy. Those 10 minutes felt like an eternity. I desperately wanted the tube out, but couldn't speak or do anything while my mouth was being forced open by a plastic funnel. It held the tube in place, and didn't allow me to bite down. I was asked to swallow repeatedly with a numb throat as the half-inch thick cord was gently fed down my throat, through the esophagus, and then into the stomach. The tube was lodged so deep, I gagged continuously.

Finally, the doctor pulled out the tube, enabling me to breathe normally again. My nerves calmed and my muscles relaxed. The constant gagging caused soreness in my chest. I wanted to get out of there quickly.

The doctor did write in his notes that he was unable to go further into the stomach because I was too nervous. I don't think the continuous gagging helped him much either. It felt like my guts wanted to jump out of my mouth. How could it be easy for the doctors to properly administer this test? I found out in later years that tranquilizers could be taken prior to the test. Thanks.

The nurse let me rest on a bed in another room as I waited for the results. It was clear to her that I was a little groggy and tired from the stress of the test. The room was noisy and hectic with doctors and nurses doing rounds.

Mariano came to see me, and we waited for the doctor. My husband was subdued, asking only how the test had gone.

"I gagged the entire time."

I was dubious about the whole procedure. Maybe it was denial, trying to convince myself that the problem was so small, it was undetectable. I felt I was wasting my time with these terrible tests. Cancer never entered my mind.

The doctor, a short Vietnamese man in a tan polo-style T-Shirt, came over to the bed and blurted out, with no preamble, that I had a tumour. And that it had to be removed.

He was nervous. This made me nervous too. I can't imagine too many patients being friendly with him or asking further details. His job was probably so unpleasant, it had affected his personality.

I only learned 11 years later that Mariano knew about the tumour before the doctor told me. The doctor had talked to him in the waiting room while I was being transferred to recovery. That explained his silence.

It was shocking to hear that he had kept that from me, but I wasn't angry. I wonder what else I don't know that doctors have told him. What other important moments during that time don't I remember? According to family and friends, I've forgotten many things that were said to me during that period.

I didn't know what to say or do after the doctor's announcement. Is he even speaking to the right patient? We listened for instructions. Well, Mariano listened mostly.

"I already scheduled an appointment with a general surgeon. He will also give you the pathology results

that was churning inside. All aspects of my life became mechanical, handling only what was imperative to address the cancer. Not being present was a blessing. The body's natural protection against stress helped me avoid bearing the pain of it all.

I can't remember where Mariano and his mother were at that point. I could only see in front of me... my parents struggling with what they had just learned.

My three older sisters were at work. I called each of them with the pathology results, but the only conversation I remember was with Susy. It didn't even dawn on me that it may not be a good idea for them to drive after hearing the news. Mary worked close by and arrived within minutes. I laugh now when I think about what she said to me as she sat around the table with my mother, my mother-in-law, and me.

"Just give me a minute, and then..." The gist of her unfinished thought, as she gestured helplessly with her hand, was that she would be strong for me once she could digest what was happening.

My oldest sister Lisa arrived soon after, since she had already finished work and was in the car driving home from Old Montreal when she heard.

The details of that day are a blur. Bits and pieces come back, but not in chronological order. Asking my family what they remember about that day is futile, as their recollections are foggy as well. My sister Mary, second in line, said that once the pathology results were revealed, things moved quickly. Ironically for me, the process was grueling and slow and seemingly endless.

Susy, 13 months older than I, stayed at work for quite some time because she was physically unable to drive after hearing the news. "Don't panic," I told her. Susy's typical reaction in a crisis is panic. Unable to process my terrible news, she passed the telephone to her colleague.

After I asked her colleague to put Susy back on the line, I tried to sound strong. "Don't worry, they will operate to remove it."

She recently admitted that after she was able to drive to my parents' house, she first stopped by the local church to pray.

Lisa's children, Claudia and Ricky, were old enough to understand the gravity of my illness. Claudia was with the man who would eventually become her husband when her mom called her. She was at his house crying for about an hour, then headed over later that afternoon, where we were all still sitting around the table. She also picked up a rosary at Notre-Dame Basilica one day after her university class, and had it blessed for me. Ricky remembers the street corner he was on, waiting for the bus after his classes ended at the local high school. He and his sister were heartbroken.

When Ricky recently told me he remembered where he was when he heard the news, I realized how bad news gets embedded in the body. We don't always remember details, but some stand out.

Human nature connects important events in our life – good and bad -- with places, things, even music. A song can remind us of high school events or moments with a partner. A landmark can recall images of a tragedy. This happens to me all the time, mostly with good memories. And the older, less pleasant memories have become just memories, much less traumatizing than initially. Still, driving by the hospital certain songs and places rise up, chasing away happier memories.

Mary's children were much younger. Sabrina was seven and Marco two, so they didn't have much comprehension of what was going on with me.

Should I have walked out? Maybe I should have slapped his face for being so cold. I suppose he thought he was being truthful.

I did wake from the test, but I never made issue with the possibility of death on the table. When I entered the doctor's low-lit office later on (Mariano remembers the room being bright), both Mariano and the specialist appeared discouraged. Mariano could barely look at me, and didn't say a word. He didn't even ask me how I was feeling, but the look on his face suggested it really didn't matter. My eyebrows rose with curiosity, but I didn't ask any questions. I read my death sentence in my husband's face.

The doctor looked right in my eye. "If you have something to do, then do it," he said quickly. No preface.

Would you be able to finish that meeting? I certainly couldn't. My mind floated away from my body again. I haven't the slightest idea what else was said, but those words are stamped into my memory for life.

Three or four years later, Mariano told me that this specialist had given me only one or three months to live. Mariano is a history buff with a great memory for facts, but this detail wasn't easy for him to recount. The doctor warned him before I came in that the prognosis was poor. "Spend the best time with her, and do what you can together."

"Oh my God... what did you say to that?" I asked.

"I thought he was mistaken. I told him it had to be more time than one to three months."

Years had passed when Mariano told me this. As far as my tests showed, I was in remission. My body proved the doctor wrong. My life seemed to be safe, for now. But when I hear the doctors' prognoses, I realize how blessed I am.

That doctor shared his negative prognosis without

apparent burden. Maybe he only sees patients when things are advanced. Mariano must have had a strenuous time deciding whether to share this sickening news with me. I think that had I really had only a few months left, I would want to know it and say my goodbyes.

In 2014, I read the specialist's results that he shared with my surgeon. "Esophageal Adenocarcinoma, Stage T3 with celiac metastasis, Grade 2."

Esophageal cancer, I have since learned, is more dangerous than stomach cancer. This doctor said I had esophageal cancer, but my surgeon told me otherwise.

During one of my visits with the surgeon a few years into remission, he tried to get me to understand that it began in the stomach and not in the esophagus. This distinction was significant regarding expected results.

One summer after my ordeal, my surgeon invited me to his annual golf fundraiser. My husband and I skipped the golf, but attended the dinner. Mariano and I were seated with the surgeon's brothers and another patient. The surgeon's wife sat with us briefly after the speeches, and she seemed just as sweet. It was a lovely evening. There was overwhelming support from the room.

During my surgeon's speech, he thanked the companies and guests for their contributions, and provided information about new research. He became emotional about one of his patients who had recently died from esophageal cancer. His humanity touched and reassured me. Doctors are just as emotional as we are, although they train themselves to subdue it in professional circumstances.

The contradiction between their endoscopy reports is irrelevant now. I am happy that the specialist was incorrect. The outcome is what matters.

With such a dismal prognosis, my survival re-

large like her father's. Her nose... a little from both. She is a beautiful girl.

Regardless of the features she inherited from her father, my cousins call her "little Patricia," after me. It makes me smile even when strangers link us. I just hope she did not inherit the health concerns I've battled throughout my life.

It was tough to tell my friends that I had cancer. I had lunch with Annette and another friend named Lina (not my colleague) regularly downtown, since we all worked in close vicinity. I told them in person. They were sad, of course, and wished me well. Annette, a longtime friend and colleague from a prior workplace, averted her eyes. "Oh, my good friend," she said, and then went speechless.

Gradually, my family and friends became aware of the devastating news, mostly circulated by my family. Medical tests, appointments, and home and work arrangements didn't allow me time to contact everyone, but my family kept me apprised of well wishes.

One day I asked Howard, "How do I get a will done quickly?" It turns out that a handwritten will is as good as one prepared by a notary, but much would be frozen until it could be notarized and homologated or approved by the court. That would mean a much higher cost to legalize my wishes. At that point, handwritten details were all I could or would take time for. Money was not a concern in what seemed like my final weeks. I just needed to organize the important issues if something were to happen to me.

So during my last couple of days at work, I attempted to write my Will. With my knee surgery, building our home, and having our daughter all coinciding, we never put serious thought into a will. We certainly didn't expect to need it so soon after the marriage.

Sitting in the food court eating my tray lunch, I began writing, *I, Patricia Rodi, being of sound mind, hereby declare this to be my final Will and Testament*... I noted my assets and how I wanted them divided, set instructions regarding my daughter and who would become her legal guardians – who was I kidding?! I had to stop because tears blurred my vision, as though I was wearing someone else's prescription glasses. I was too embarrassed to look up from the paper. The thin napkins handed to me with my tray were shredding from blowing my nose repeatedly.

I couldn't tell if the people around me, also on lunch break, noticed I was crying. As an observer-type, I would have asked myself if that person was writing a goodbye letter or something. Who would imagine it was a legal document about her death?

Never write your Will when you're on your deathbed. Try to handle these legal issues early in life, when you're of clear mind.

A few nights later, I tried to distribute the assets and investments I held among my husband, daughter, and family. My biggest concern was that since Isabella was only one year old, I felt she needed a mother figure to look after her.

Mariano and I agreed that if I were to die, my parents could move in permanently. Since he works five days a week, my mother could care for her as a mother should.

# Chapter 4

# My Big Day

*The night before I entered the hospital for surgery, a family friend invited a local priest to my house to sit with me and my family.*

I have come to believe that old cliché that things happen for a reason. Looking back, I have to admit that my health issues over the years prepared me for cancer. I've worn eye glasses since the second grade (I can remember the school nurse holding out a letter, "Take this to your parents.") I was in the fifth grade, age ten, when the ophthalmologist showed me how to put on contact lenses. A major car accident at the age of 23 left me with a protrusion on the head the size and colour of an eggplant, broken ribs and arm, and severe back pain. A few years after the crash, I was hospitalized for pneumonia, and later diagnosed with asthma. A skating fall in January of 2001 required surgery to reattach the posterior knee ligament in my left leg. And according to my stomach tumour pathology report, tumours were growing at the time of the knee injury, and likely as far back as 1998, the year I met my husband.

The skating accident happened only three months after my wedding. That was my first experience with general anesthesia. Prior to the knee surgery, I was scared of anesthesia. It can kill you. Fatalities are rare, but there is a possibility that you won't wake up from it (where have I heard that before?) When I heard I would undergo major surgery for cancer, I had no fear of being put to sleep.

Shortly after my mother's sister died from Leukemia in 1988, I had dreamt about her. She stood a few feet away from me, wearing a white bell-style coat. The feeling the dream gave me was that she was well, and that she would always be close to us. She didn't need to speak. I can still see the beautiful woman who remains in my heart.

Some time after that dream, I had a nightmare about the apartment upstairs from my parents' house in Saint-Leonard. I was in the kitchen of the apartment with someone else (I am not sure who) and we were squatting in front of the counter in the dark. The room was on fire and a large, dark figure shielded us from the flames with her big arms and body. We feared the fire, but felt the protection. I woke from the dream after hearing a sound. The source of the sound was near my bed. Too tired to be curious, I fell asleep again.

Getting out of bed the next morning, I felt something under my foot. A religious pin that I had been keeping in the top drawer of my nightstand had fallen. The pin had a picture of Archangel Michael, leader of the heavenly body of angels. He plays an important role in the Book of Revelations, the last book of the New Testament. He defeats a dragon and tosses him into the abyss.

I hadn't touched that pin and it had never fallen before. I took it as an omen. My aunt, I felt, was the protector – my angel. I should not be afraid, my dreams were saying. An angel would watch over me.

September 28 was fast approaching, and that past summer was eventful, to say the least. My Dad had turned eighty a short time before my diagnosis. We celebrated his milestone by renting a large cabin up north that could accommodate all fifteen of us.

My Dad's wish for his birthday was fulfilled. He loves just being with his family. He's at the age when fancy parties don't appeal to him.

That weekend the weather was great. The chalet in Mont Tremblant Park offered bedrooms for each couple. Mary's children slept on the large sofa bed in the living room. Mariano, Isabella, and I shared a room with bunk beds that I would never dream of sleeping on again. My young daughter and I shared the bottom bunk to help distribute the weight on what seemed like an unstable set up. The large, private master bedroom in which my parents slept was on the second floor. The kitchen was average size, but too small for all the cooks in the family. A wooden dining table accommodated most of us. We had a fireplace that wasn't needed in August, but added ambiance, regardless of the furnishings.

We spent some time walking the mountain area where people ski in the winter. My dad and brothers-in-law enjoyed the view from our cabin balcony as others cooked, set the table, and watched the children sing the Italian songs my parents loved. We filmed the weekend, so we could show the children their talents when they got older.

We brought lasagna for dinner and breakfast items. The crowded kitchen created a feast for the meals we shared there. In our family, it's always about food. Pictures from my photo albums reminded me of the one dinner we shared at a local family restaurant. We all sang happy birthday as my Dad blew the candle on a dessert we ordered.

When we watched that video after my bout with cancer, I noticed that my skin tone had changed. I was dark by nature, more so than my sisters. That olive tone had turned dull and yellowish from the cancer. I looked ill. None of us had perceived the change in my skin colour as negative, even though I was in the process of testing for that bleeding incident. Everyone was accustomed to my colour being different. My oldest brother-in-law, Ralph, used to joke I was adopted.

We went apple picking on the Saturday prior to my operation. I wasn't in the mood to pick apples, and remember just wanting to relax that day. Somehow, fruit picking seemed unimportant compared to spending the day with my family.

I brought a blanket and lay in the grass by the trees, close to where my family was filling the plastic bags with McIntosh and Cortlands. I didn't want them to be out of sight. But I also needed some time alone to think about what was happening.

My energy level was decreasing. My surgeon had told me that following the operation, I could return to work after two months or so. During our meetings, I was told that chemo and radiation were not an absolute part of the plan. The operation was no guarantee of success, and that full protocol would follow only if the surgery worked out.

Was the prognosis so grim that I would not work again? This did not cross my mind, but now I am curious about what the medical team thought about the probability of success.

That same weekend before surgery, family and friends gathered at my house. A dear friend of my mother, who has since died from cancer, asked our local priest to come and offer his blessing.

We all prayed with the priest, and then he chatted with us for a while. He asked me if we could speak privately. "Sometimes," he said, "we must leave our life in God's hands, and trust that our faith will help us through."

The more he spoke, the more convinced I was ready to put my life in the hands of a stranger, my surgeon. The priest also asked me about my life and my faith.

A sense of peace overcame me. The priest's words suggested that I wouldn't be alone during my most trying time. God was a strong presence in my life. But this priest, who was only a man and who later had his own health problems, was the one who helped me find my courage.

I asked my mom to come and live with me once I returned from the hospital. The surgeon had told me that I'd stay in the hospital for about 10 days, so it seemed futile, in my mother's eyes, to plan that far in advance. She said she would see how things were.

There wasn't a doubt that she would be there for me, for my daughter, to help out at home while I recovered. But she seemed unable to commit to a long-term plan. Did she know something I did not? I needed reassurance that everything would be in place by the time I returned home. But my family has shown me that they will always be there to take care of us.

To ensure that my mother and father would be comfortable, I asked her to arrange for her spare bed to be brought over while I was in the hospital. She agreed.

Monday, September 27, 2004, I entered the hospital as they had instructed. When my surgeon came to see me later that afternoon, I pointed to the frame with my daughter's pictures. "Save me for her."

In my semi-private room, I made a final review of my will. I included personalized messages to Mariano, Isabella, my parents, siblings, and nieces and nephews. I was much less emotional that day as I wrote, then I tucked the will away in my purse. No one knew I had written it, but it would certainly be found if something went wrong.

I was oblivious to the baby-blue-coloured walls in the room, and the neighbour that went about her business in the bed next to me. Though only a dull-beige curtain separated us, I felt I was alone.

That evening, I began the preparation for surgery. I was handed a full glass of salt water to clean out my digestive system. You can imagine how that went.

I threw up after drinking about half of the glass. I rinsed my mouth at the washroom sink.

Mariano called the nurse to let her know that I had vomited and asked if I still needed to drink more.

She stood there, uncaring and upset, "if you don't drink the rest of it, the doctor will not operate tomorrow."

By the end of the long evening, I had forced down the rest of it. My feces turned clear as the ocean.

At midnight the nurse told my husband to leave.

I don't remember whether I slept well that night. I didn't feel like I was tossing and turning all night. In retrospect, there wasn't any fear at that point, since I had made the decision to put my life in God's hands – and the surgeon's. I felt safe and calm – probably due to that dazed, shocked mode that carried me through the experience. Without a clue of what was to come, I was prepared to find out.

Sometime during the very early morning of September 28, an orderly came into the room and told me he would take me to the operating room in the basement. He said I should leave my prescription glasses in my room, so they would not get lost. The entire ride was blurry. I abhor that insecurity of near blindness. My severe myopia prevented me from seeing even the face of the man who was rolling my bed who knows where. I should be used to the lack of vision, but it still makes me uncomfortable in places I don't know. If I'm addressed, I will follow the voice, facial details are hazy. At home, I know where things are, so it's easier to get around.

Few thoughts went through my mind that morning. Clearly, I was anxious to know whether the cancer was operable. I would have loved to watch the surgery from a balcony like we see on television.

The attendant stopped in a small hallway near the operating room. There wasn't any natural light, only dim LEDs from the ceiling.

"Your family has come to wish you well, but then I have to get you prepped next door."

I hadn't seen my family that day, and it was comforting to know they were close to the O.R. Their love and loyalty is clear, so I knew they would be there.

My mother's fear betrayed her, and her repeated kisses and unrelenting grip of my hand made me feel connected to every part of what she had been trying so desperately to hide.

"I'll be okay. *Ti voglio bene.*"

She said she loved me.

Before I knew it, my family vanished and I was wheeled into the large operating room. The room was bright and cold. The staff were extremely friendly, but only a few spoke to me. Things were organized and everyone was calm.

Some of the nurses were preparing equipment and medical tools. On my right, I could see a table covered in blue sheets. Atop lay the cutting instruments, including the scalpel that would slice me open. It was just as well I couldn't see. People's faces, hair, and hands were covered.

The anesthesiologist approached to explain her procedure. "Good morning. I am Doctor…" She asked me to confirm my name.

Remembering my knee surgery, I laughed when she told me to begin counting to 100. I barely recall saying number three. As my eyes began to close, I entered a calm that lasted a second before plunging into a drug-induced sleep.

One, tw... and I'm out. My job was done. I wonder at what point the surgeon walked in. The casual greetings amongst him and the assistants surely included a joke or two. Maybe music played in the background. It would be a long day for him, with an investigation and the operation on the same day.

My niece, Claudia, then in university, stayed home that day with a good family friend, to take care of Isabella and Marco. My husband, mother, sisters, and oldest brother-in-law, Ralph - who's more like the brother I never had – sat impatiently in the hospital waiting room. We had been told that the longer they were left to wait, the better the news could be. My surgeon explained that, once he completed the physical investigation – which would take three or four hours, he would only put me through the risky surgery if he knew he could remove all the cancer. He told my family that if he didn't come out by noon, that meant he would be able to do the surgery. My sister Mary told me later that they were panicking, hoping he would not appear.

Susy later told me that they all visited the chapel to pray that morning. That moved me, but I hated the thought of their anguish. Mariano remained in the waiting room. He is not so religious, but I imagine he wanted to be there for the doctor.

Lisa said they kept watching everyone who came out of the O.R., anxious about whether they would approach our family. By noon, some of the fear subsided, but they were still worried about the results.

Late that afternoon, the surgeon emerged in his scrubs. He approached Mariano, carrying a notepad and pen. He liked to draw pictures to explain procedures.

My family crowded in, watching and listening. The surgeon provided details of the successful operation. He explained that tumours were all over the bottom of the stomach as well - which we hadn't known - so he had to remove the entire stomach, as well as about one-third of the esophagus. Only one cut on the front torso had to be made for a total gastrectomy, so he'd been able to discard the plan to also cut a long curve down my back. I was under the knife for eight hours in total.

Although I'd lost my entire stomach, I feel it was the best result. It meant the cancer would not spread, as the stomach lining can hide potentially threatening cancer cells. Had the surgeon missed a single malignant cell, the surgery would have been for nothing.

The surgeon explained the "Roux-en-Y" procedure, where the small intestine gets pulled up and connected to the remaining esophagus. The duodenum is also reattached to the small intestine. Thirteen lymph nodes were also removed, of which only three were cancerous.

The surgeon had initially told me that he would remove only the upper part of my stomach, which was infested with tumours, as well as part of the esophagus. They always remove a little more, to be safe. Then he would lift my intestine and connect the remaining stomach to the esophagus near my shoulder. I would have had a scar down my middle – starting under the rib cage and extending to below the belly button, as I do now. On my back there would be a large quarter-moon design.

I laugh at the reaction I might have gotten from people who would hear me say, "I have a stomach ache," and I'd place my hand to my shoulder.

My sisters re-explained the situation to my mother, who was having trouble following.

They poured out their thanks and gratitude. "When can we see her?"

Writing this now makes me cry. I can't imagine what relief they must have felt. Once I was drugged, I did not worry. I forgot about the investigation and the resulting decision of whether to operate. For my family, the ordeal was much harder.

My dad, who was at Lisa's house with Claudia, received updates throughout the day. He had not been told that the entire stomach was removed. I don't know why my sisters would think having part of my stomach removed would be less traumatizing for him. He is still unaware of this fact today.

The first time I remember opening my eyes, I didn't feel a thing. For all I knew, I was missing more than my stomach. I was still under the effects of the epidural.

I realized I was in a room that appeared different each time I awakened. It was unclear how much time had elapsed between each snooze, and what time of day it was. Without my contact lenses or glasses, my vision was still a blur. The lighting was so dim, I thought it was night. I could tell I was alone. It felt peaceful; not at all like being in a hospital. I was comfortable and pain-free.

For a few moments, I felt lonely and intimidated – almost frightened by the emptiness around me. I stared at the ceiling, then toward the light on the right, trying to become aware of where I was. The feel-good medication must have had something to do with my lack of concern at that point.

That quiet room was Intensive Care – the place you rest in the hours immediately following important surgeries.

The light was coming from the rectangular-shaped window connecting the next room. I had imagined it was a viewing room for nurses, but my husband informed me that it was an operating room.

Again I awakened, but this time there was a shape hovering by my bed. It was the surgeon. He put his hand over mine - a real gentleman - happy he saved another life. "We did it." He was humble, and emotional.

I could only smile, feeling happy, even though I'd been through so much. What a miracle to receive a second chance. I forced a mumble through the tubes down my nose and throat, "Merci." Thank you.

Nothing else needed to be said. Before he could even walk out the door, I was asleep.

He left me in the hands of a trusted colleague and went on holiday.

Later that evening, my husband's brother, Mike, and a friend of Susy's came by the hospital. As I opened my eyes again, Mariano and Mike stood by my bed, staring mutely, waiting for a sign of life. I could see my brother-in-law's smile. He was over six feet tall, fair-skinned, with short razored hair on his head.

The light from the glass behind them helped me recognize their silhouettes. You would never think they were siblings given their shapes and colouring. My husband took after his mother, and Mike, his father.

Mariano is about five foot six, with full, unshaved black hair. He didn't play sports much, but tells me he occasionally did the street hockey thing and played soccer for a short time in his early teens. He ice skates really well. Mike loved golf, hockey, and hunting – taking week-long trips into the wilderness.

Ralph told me recently that he, my mother, and sisters were first at my bedside in intensive care. I don't remember seeing them, but he said I was awake, and had signaled two thumbs up.

The next day or so, I was in a more populated recovery area on another floor, where more than immediate family was allowed. I remember telling the nurse that the tubes hurt, and finally they pulled them out of my nose, leaving my throat on fire and my voice hoarse for days. The nurses made sure the epidural took care of all other pain. I wouldn't say it was easy, but so far, I was content.

Soon I had my first new visitors. I can imagine family and friends were awaiting news about the surgery. Having been so involved with my own drama, I had forgotten about the world. It was heartwarming to find so many people remembering me.

My cousin – once removed, Nick and his wife Tanya, stood at the end of the bed. What a sweet gesture, I thought. Nick and I are the same age, and we share fun childhood memories with all our cousins. Although as adults we had our own lives, we kept in touch. Seeing him that day was very moving.

Claudia told me that she had called Gerry to let him know the operation went well – as I had asked her to do. She said he wanted to visit. I was thrilled to see him for those few minutes and thank him again for finding the surgeon.

Several weeks later, Gerry told me how happy he was that he had received that phone call. He had split up with his wife, and that day was the first wedding anniversary they faced apart.

Eventually, I settled into a semi-private room on yet another floor, beside a window – which I prefer. I still had no pain with the epidural in full force. Recovery was going well, but I became a little bored because I couldn't move. I did not like lying around, but the medication lulled me in and out of sleep for the first days.

The cushion they had given me to press against my belly was of little use as I barely coughed or sneezed. It was as if my body had left on vacation with the surgeon. If the occasional sneeze or cough came, it was so quick that I had no time to grab the cushion. It felt like my stitches were ripping open, but there was never any damage. The catheter took care of my urine that first week – the epidural kept my torso, hips, and legs numb.

My sisters and mother came every day, and they brought my father once I started to look better.

Susy took her vacation from work so she could be there during my second week at the hospital, when I needed more attention. She and my mother visited during the day. Susy always made sure my telephone was disinfected and my tray table organized. Actually, she was a little obsessive about it. It didn't make a difference to me at the time due to my inactivity, but it's good to keep a hospital room clean.

I don't remember each visit, but friends, family, and colleagues came by the hospital to spend time with me. They even brought gifts. I'm always surprised when I know people are thinking of me. Their presence was a welcome gift.

My husband passed by the hospital after work. As soon as he'd arrive, he'd tell me he was going for a bite, which bothered me, because I could not join him.

The first weekend, my parents and sisters and their families were at the hospital when dinner hour came. I heard them whispering options of where they could go and eat.

"Why don't you just pick up something and have it here?" I asked.

It felt really nice to have them all there together, and I didn't want them to leave. "You could get smoked meat sandwiches or roast chicken. It's alright with me... I'll just smell it."

It was an awkward moment. I wasn't eating at that point. Hunger didn't exist yet. I missed the smell of real food.

They gave in when they saw it was what I wanted.

Back then I was receiving 1,200 calories daily through the intestinal tube in my belly. The surgeon connected a jejunostomy (or J-Tube), a feeding tube surgically inserted during the gastrectomy into my intestine and protruding from the middle of the belly. A feeding bag hung on a pole beside me. I would need it until I was able to ingest food orally. I had lost a lot of weight and also muscle mass due to bed rest, but I certainly did not feel hungry.

Overnight, *living to eat* (my passion for food) turned into *eating to live*. I would have to adapt to my cut and stitched anatomy quickly to ensure a healthy weight going forward.

The BBQ chicken and fries that my brothers-in-law picked up for everyone smelled good, stirring memories of late-night takeout of extra pepperoni pizza with my sisters when they lived upstairs from my parents in the apartment complex my parents owned. Now the mouth-watering aroma of BBQ chicken also helped mask the chemical cleaner that pervaded that hospital setting.

I had a lifelong passion for food and cooking. Gourmet and international cuisines were more exotic to me than the Italian dishes I'd grown up with. Mariano and I love Asian cuisine in particular, so I learned to make Maki rolls, Chinese dishes, and Peking Duck. Oh, how I miss those flavours already.

Since my family spent so much time at the hospital, they got to know the patients sharing my room. Swapping stories with other patients and their family members was a great pastime for us all.

Patients were coming and going in the bed next to me. Some were in critical state. I was less aware of the goings on compared to my family, especially during the first week.

In the second week, during naps, I began having nightmares about my daughter. They were awfully graphic and kept repeating, with the details growing worse. Horrible things would happen to her. She was caught in a fire, or would fall from a height. I couldn't help her, or get to her. I felt helpless in the dreams, and guilty afterwards for dreaming them. The fear was traumatizing. After six or seven nightmares, I told the nurse that I wasn't able to tolerate it anymore.

She stared at me blankly for a moment, and then explained that the epidural could be causing anxiety. She said she'd reduce it. The nightmares subsided soon after that.

Eventually, the epidural was replaced with oral painkillers. The skin on my torso still felt numb, and I couldn't imagine what was going on inside where my stomach used to be. I don't remember any pain following the surgery. I wondered whether I would feel something after the drug regimen ended and the numbness stopped.

My knee surgery three years earlier had been excruciating. They put me under general anesthesia not once, but twice. The second time was to force my leg straight and set a full-leg cast. I couldn't get enough painkillers after waking that time.

The nurse brought me a special tube to strengthen my breathing. It was a simple, plastic thing called an incentive spirometer, with markers to verify improvement. Inside was a small yellow piston that moved as I blew into the top. It was supposed to facilitate secretions and strengthen breathing, which was weak following surgery. I had to practise breathing with it ten times every hour for several days. They even made me take it home.

During the second week, the extent of my weight loss became apparent. I had lost five pounds earlier that summer from trying *The South Beach Diet*. Not that I was overweight, but I wanted to get healthier. What I would give to take those pounds back. Another five pounds melted away prior to the operation, and 10 more while I lay in bed in the hospital. From 140 pounds, I was now

120, and losing pounds daily from bedrest and a liquid diet. Within the next few weeks, I dipped down to 94 pounds. The feeding tube helped, but only to maintain weight, not to gain it.

My blood work kept showing anemia, so the nurses monitored it daily, at an hour when I just wanted to sleep. When the doctor requested that I get out of bed and walk, I was so weak, I could barely comply.

The nurse lowered the bed rail, and stayed with me as I tried to sit up. I managed to turn my body, and let my legs hang from the side of the bed like limp ropes. The nurse watched to see if I could stand on my own.

My head was in a whirlwind. I attempted to walk by the bed, but the dizziness worsened. My vision started to tunnel and I collapsed into a chair by the wall. The nurse didn't intervene.

She was staring at my chart, not attending to me. My head was still, now, but the room continued to spin. My head was so heavy, I could barely hold it up. It felt like it was filled with liquid, and someone was shaking it like a snow globe. My ears were blocked, and all the sounds from the corridor boomed in my head. Even my voice sounded distant. After sitting for several minutes, the strange feeling faded.

The nurse helped me back into bed. "I'll have to speak to your doctor about this," she said. Then she disappeared into the hallway.

The doctor said I needed blood. That frightened me, because we'd had trouble a few years ago in Quebec with blood infected with HIV and hepatitis. "I don't know if I want to do that," I said.

The nurse assured me the blood was carefully tested and would make a big and positive difference. "You lost quite a bit of blood during the operation."

Blood tests revealed that I had severe anemia, which was why I couldn't stand up.

"I'll let you know tomorrow," I said.

She nodded, her eyes urging me to agree to a transfusion.

How awful it would be if I rid myself of the cancer only to catch a disease from someone else's blood. I ought to have kept Isabella's umbilical cord. Umbilical cords can be used to make your own blood. But I'd had cancer during my pregnancy, so perhaps I would have been barred from using the umbilical cord in this way. The new blood would be healthy, but it might also contain the potential for generating new cancer. I am no scientist, but my imagination began working overtime.

The next day, I still couldn't get out of bed, so I agreed to a transfusion, which was administered immediately. The nurse hooked me up to an IV unit, and for two hours, a stranger's blood entered my veins...a stranger with a generous heart.

The next morning, I couldn't believe the burst of energy. I left my bed without any problem.

A couple of months before my cancer diagnosis, I was having lunch at a downtown food court. As I was heading back to the office, I walked past an area where people were lying on beds and drinking orange juice. There were IVs next to each bed, and bags filling with blood. I considered donating. I asked a Red Cross organizer for a business card, and tucked it in my wallet. I wanted to help. My health was generally good, but I had started having symptoms of the cancer, and they made me hesitate. I was determined to give blood when I felt a little stronger.

Unfortunately, the diagnosis came, putting an end to that plan. Had I donated that day, would cancer have been detected? Probably not. Although they might have picked up on the anemia.

I forgot about the card and it sat in my wallet until long after my treatments. I called the clinic to see if I could donate blood if I was in remission. The answer was no.

I appreciate more than ever the importance of donating blood. Unfortunately, I doubt I will ever have the opportunity to offer the gift that was offered to me.

Ten days after surgery the doctor decided I was ready to eat orally, and my first hospital meal arrived on a plastic tray. I raised the cover and found a lump of meat, mashed potatoes from powder, and soggy vegetables from the freezer.

I am supposed to have only liquids at first. I told the nurse, and a new tray was brought. What havoc this serious error could have caused, had I eaten what was there. Mistakes happen. It's important, when you're in hospital, to be vigilant and take care of yourself.

My first meal was beef broth. I couldn't take much. For one thing I wasn't hungry, and for another, I hate beef. I began dreaming of my mom's homemade chicken soup.

Two days later they brought me the plate with a lump of meat and powdered mash again. Eating was not exactly a pleasure. I forced down some of the mash, leaving more than half on the plate. It did not make me sick, even after more than an hour.

I hadn't the slightest idea how much my body would accept. No one taught me about quantity. The nurses were unfamiliar with gastrectomy diets. The only clue I had been given was to eat smaller and more frequent meals. I guess I was supposed to figure it out on my own.

Another day, I received a roast chicken leg. I managed a few bites, but soon felt pain in my esophagus. The food was stuck, so I stopped eating after the next bite made it worse. It took a long time for the pain to subside. I wasn't up to trying to eat again. My next meal went down easier, but I had to eat slowly and chew endlessly before swallowing.

One evening during the second week in hospital, I received an amazing surprise. It was after dinner and my parents and sisters were visiting. Our family is big, so people were standing around the foot of the bed, and the others were in the hallway, or else visiting with my neighbour in the next bed.

From the doorway, I heard voices. I couldn't see because a curtain surrounded my bed. The voices grew louder. My neighbour's visitors on the other side of the curtain sounded cheerful.

The mystery was solved when Mariano walked in carrying our little girl in his arms. How unexpected and wonderful. With the challenges of the last two weeks, I had all but forgotten who I was – the mother of a beautiful little girl. I sat up, throwing off the blankets. My arms went out to her.

She was wearing a hospital mask, which confused me. I longed to hold her, but I knew I wasn't ready. The skin on my torso was still raw. Mariano held her in his arms near the end of the bed. I threw myself forward to kiss her.

She stared hard at me, horrified, as if she did not fully recognize me.

I had not realized how altered I was until my little girl's visit. The tube from my intestine was hidden by my blue hospital gown, and no tubes or IVs were connected to me at that point, but I was clearly not the mother I had been before leaving for the hospital.

I wish I could comfort her. She just kept staring at me, not saying a word.

"Why is she wearing a mask?" I finally managed to ask.

"She has a cold, and we wanted to make sure she doesn't infect you."

"Oh, Sweetie. Are you all right?" I asked her. But again, Mariano had to step in as her spokesman.

"She'll be okay. We gave her some medicine."

"She doesn't like the mask. If she's congested, she's probably having trouble breathing with it. She looks horrified." My eyes turned back to Isabella. "I love you…" I blurted out, unable to reassure her through hugs or the touch that young children need and crave. I smiled and held her ghostly gaze.

But that gaze was disturbing. She looked dazed, almost drugged. Was it the cold medication? She looked at me, barely blinking. I yearned to hold her in my arms.

My family, concerned about Isabella's cold, wouldn't let me touch her. My own pain medication made me docile, and I went along with it. Isabella stayed masked the whole visit, encased in Mariano's arms. I was happy beyond words to have her there, but seconds later, it seemed, Mariano left to take her home. He had defied my family's wishes to bring her that night, I learned much later. That was fine by me.

As I became stronger, I met Isabella and my husband in the first floor lobby. My sister took me down in a wheelchair, so I could spend more time with my daughter, who was feeling better. As I began sleeping less, I missed her more. I couldn't wait to leave the hospital and get home to her.

Those brief visits with Isabella reminded me how blessed I was, and reinforced my will to heal and to live.

Two weeks is a huge period to be absent in the life of a child. And it's very long for a mother as well. Time had stopped. There was no yesterday and certainly no tomorrow in those first days in the hospital. Just a very demanding and busy present moment. Doctors, tests, and predictions of imminent death. This was my life now, and it had turned my life as a mother upside down.

Nearing the end of my stay, the industrial-sized staples that held my skin together were removed. A young nurse came into my room and explained that it would not be painful. She said she would try to remove the metal staples with the large tweezers she held in her hand – a tool that looked more like something she had found in her garage.

She seemed nervous, but I wasn't about to shake things up.

She raised my bed to a half-sitting position, and began to pinch the first staple with the tweezers. She shifted it left to right, gently and slowly, attempting to slide it away from my skin. She described her actions, as though this would make me less nervous. Her description matched her actions, keeping my fear at bay.

My hands rose to my mouth just in case, and I held my breath with each pull. My eyes shifted from her to the ceiling each time she started on the next staple. They were as wide and almost as thick as a nickel, so I thought for sure it would hurt as they left my skin.

After a few minutes, she casually let slip that it was her first time doing this.

Somehow, we got through the ordeal.

# Chapter 5

# Coming Home

*When you have cancer, it's natural for people to be uncomfortable around you.*

The operation was successful, and at last I was going home. As excited as I was to get out of the hospital, I knew it would take a while to return to anything like a normal life. But I was not thinking ahead.

We had waited some time for my walking papers, so when I told Mariano I wanted to say goodbye to the nurses, he told me to be quick. La famiglia was waiting at home. The goodbyes done, Mariano wheeled me in a hospital wheelchair to the accounting department, to check out. Hopefully, I would never return to this hotel again.

I was tired. I had moved about a lot that day. Even though Mariano did most of the work, getting dressed and gathering my things took huge amounts of effort. My ability to move and bend was limited.

Mariano remembers driving home slowly, because the numerous potholes caused pain in my abdomen. The nurse told me to take home the coughing cushion. I kept it pressed against my belly during the ride. Mariano and I barely spoke, so we could concentrate on avoiding all the holes.

Finally, we approached our house in Rivière-des-Prairies ("RDP"), one of the many Montreal suburban boroughs. I was eager to be in my own space again, my new home, away from the hospital. Most of all, I wanted to see Isabella.

Although it was mid-October, it was warm and sunny. There were so many nice days that fall while I was fighting for my life. It was as if the sun was trying to encourage me.

My family was congregated at our home, getting it ready for my return. We arrived past one thirty. As Mariano unlocked our front door, my mother and Lisa were right behind it. The warm welcome sent chills through me, and my beautiful daughter ran straight into my arms.

With some caution, I knelt and hugged her. I told her I had missed her. How could I expect her to understand what was going on, and why I had been away for so long? She hadn't forgotten me. That was clear. It felt incredible to hold her again, even though I was unable to pick her up.

I moved slowly for some time. My torso was intimidating for all of us. People couldn't guess at the tenderness of my skin, but they were careful around me. My family avoided hugging me more than they wanted to.

As numb as my chest and belly were, my skin there was sensitive to the touch. The fabrics I wore heightened the awkward sensation. I still had the J-Tube attached, and it left a bump through my shirt. Today, when any one touches my abdomen it feels tender. Without any stomach, I have an emptiness inside that makes me feel fragile.

My nephew and brother-in-law play-fight with me

sometimes. When they reach their arms around me from behind to pick me up, it does not feel good. The area below the ribs is sunken, and it feels really strange when pressure is applied there.

A feast was laid out on the metal table my parents had given us to use until we bought our own dining-room set. We hadn't bought all our furniture yet. Isabella's bedroom set was new, but we had several more rooms to fill now that we were out of the apartment.

The dining room in our house opens into the living room, offering lots of space. The swimming six-foot metal table was groaning with pastry-bought pizza, cold cuts, fresh panini, homemade giardiniera, and a cheese and olive platter. For the first time in my life, I felt wary of food. There was no hunger or even comfort at the sight of it. In fact, there was fear without a medical professional to help me if something went wrong.

Even before the operation, when I was having esophageal pain, food was problematic. Now, it assumed the level of threat.

"Do you want me to make you a plate?" my sister Lisa asked.

I shook my head. "I only just started eating solids. This is way too complicated for me."

It hit me that perhaps I would never again be able to splurge when it came to eating. It was a whole new world. I felt like an infant being fed Pablum for the first time. I had to start at the beginning.

"But we waited, so we could have lunch together."

"Go ahead. But I really can't. I'm not hungry." I felt terrible for all the trouble they had gone through for me. But I suppose we all had to learn about my new way of eating.

Pizza, cold cuts, cheese... all complicated foods

that I hadn't yet tried. My mom offered to make me soup. They were probably famished, but didn't want to eat until I arrived.

Eating for the first time unsupervised was intimidating. The last thing I had eaten was at the hospital that morning. I did not want to risk getting ill, or blocked. Returning to the hospital was not on my menu.

Sharing meals is a big part of Italian culture. The main course is usually followed by several desserts. Normally, we would just buy Italian pastries, or my mother would bake cookies or her amazing traditional four-layer cake that had 12 eggs, a coffee-and-sweet-liquor-mix, and plenty of custard (both chocolate and vanilla). She would dust the top with icing sugar and candy sprinkles.

In 2010, my oldest brother-in-law, Ralph, was diagnosed with diabetes, so we reduced the desserts for his benefit. We continue to look for tasty sugar-free desserts, but now usually skip this part of the meal. My sister Lisa, Ralph's wife, cooks with much less salt, and they avoid sugar. He's really good at controlling his once strong sweet tooth.

Ralph's doctor initially wanted him hospitalized because his illness was so acute. When Ralph told the doctor he would take care of it, I don't know if either of them realized how well he would do. I'm both grateful and full of admiration at how he turned his life around. My life wouldn't be the same without him.

Ralph didn't tell all our family right away about his diagnosis. He had to absorb it and get into a routine. He gave up chain smoking with the help of a patch, began exercising and walking every day, and ate healthy meals to help stabilize his sugar. Within a few months, he looked healthier than I had ever seen him.

He had good reasons to fight. His oldest child, Claudia, was expecting his first grandchild. That was a strong motivation. Today, he still gets up early to walk and he eats well. He went from daily insulin and pills to just a half-pill.

# Chapter 6
# Make It Stop

*How do I survive this?*

My hand grasps the phone as I purse my lips to stop gagging. On the other end of the line is a friend checking in on me.

"Hold on," I tell her. With sweaty palms and growling in my belly, I signal my mother to take the phone. I grab the bucket that sits next to me and run to the washroom, only a few feet from the couch that has been my refuge for months.

I hope my mother figures out she should tell my friend I am too ill to finish our conversation. By now, she knows the signs of gastral distress.

The diarrhea comes with a vengeance. The vomit is mostly saliva, since I haven't been eating. The continuous gagging has made the interior incision sore. Diarrhea brings on hemorrhoids.

The days are long when all I can do is lie here, waiting for these gastric attacks. The bucket has become my best friend, and the couch, my mother. The couch and pillow provide a haven for pain and weakness. I sit and lie on the couch so much throughout my treatments, leaning on one side, that I develop shoulder and neck pain.

My chemotherapy treatments began on my daughter's second birthday, November 29, two months after my operation. I organized a small party the day before to celebrate the miracle in my life. It was a great distraction.

Would I make it to Isabella's third birthday? I did not know. Would she remember me if I left her now? Probably not.

Each birthday or Christmas that I celebrate with Isabella, I write her a letter revealing what she means to me. They are accumulating in her Christmas stocking, and I hope she'll look at them again later in life with positive reminiscences.

That second birthday or Christmas I wasn't able to honour the custom I had created on her first birthday, one year earlier. Though I felt strong on her second birthday, I must have forgotten about writing it in all the busyness of preparing her party. And I was preoccupied with the upcoming treatments.

The letters I did manage every subsequent year reflected on the past year, what I had learned about being a mother, lessons we taught each other, important events in our lives, and aspirations for the future. I also write each of my nieces and nephews special letters at Christmas.

After surgery, my mother moved in to take care of me and my family. It was a good thing, because my oncologist decided that my emaciated 110-pound body could handle chemotherapy. By then, I had lost 30 pounds. I had no idea this was just the beginning.

All my appointments were well organized by the hospital oncology department, and I simply had to follow instructions provided by the secretaries on the fourth floor of the hospital.

Mariano and I headed to the oncology blood centre down the hall for what would become routine blood tests. Each visit, the doctor reviewed the pertinent markers. Doctor visits and blood tests were scheduled prior to the treatment week, so the oncologist would have results available to determine whether doses needed adjusting.

From the waiting room, I was directed to a long narrow room where at least seven or eight blue and green reclining chairs were lined up along a 40-foot wall. They weren't the cozy chairs you would put in your family room. They were boxy, with a high back rest and covered in thick vinyl. Not as comfortable as I would have liked. I wished the surroundings were prettier, like the new lounges in some hospitals. It felt very clinical, but during the Christmas holiday, the nurses put a two-foot artificial tree on the counter, decorated with colourful ornaments and a flashing star at the top.

I often sat in the same area. But wherever I took refuge, the room always felt grim. The nurses went about their duties, trying to lighten the mood. Patients sat and stared listlessly at nothing as they received their poison. It was mostly silent and sad.

My first treatment included a lot of preparation and information sharing with the nurse assigned to my file that day.

Each time I walked in, heads would turn slightly, and I could feel the eyes on me. The impassive expressions loudly reminded me where I was. My appointments were always mid-afternoon, and I don't remember ever seeing other patients walking in after me. Chemo treatments last at least a couple of hours up to a day. Some patients had been in that room since early morning, but didn't have to return the rest of the week like I did.

I seldom recognized faces in the treatment rooms during my sessions. I couldn't help wondering how many people passed through here each week.

I don't remember seeing the others grow nauseated, whereas I had the vomit tray on my lap every visit. I also looked more sick than the others. Some people don't get nauseated with chemo. Perhaps I was susceptible, or maybe I had nausea because of the type of cancer medication I was receiving.

The gagging and nausea began the moment I'd step into my house. Perhaps the anti-nausea medications they doped me with during the treatment kept me from vomiting all over their furniture and floor. It would certainly be discouraging to watch patients vomit on top of receiving the treatments for hours on end at the clinic.

Following each treatment, I couldn't get home fast enough. I would get a blanket, a bucket, and climb on the couch. I was too tired to go upstairs to bed, and besides, I wanted to be around Isabella.

The first two treatments were awful. If each treatment was so rough, was it worth the risk? Chemotherapy can actually kill you. The things that my body went through those first six or seven months made me wonder if I would make it past the preventative measures stage.

After a few days following treatment, all the side effects descended at once. I vomited with painful mouth sores that made my gums swell. It was difficult to stay hydrated. Hemorrhoids made it difficult to sit. Exhaustion and weakness made it more difficult to reach for the bucket and run to the washroom.

It was out of control. How can a starving, weakened body endure such hardship? I got weaker. And then the fever began.

Fever was the one thing the nurses warned me about. I was to go to the emergency the moment my temperature rose. So I called the ambulance, and after some inquisition, they took me to my treating hospital, where I was placed in isolation. This period following chemotherapy injections is called neutropenia. The body becomes more susceptible to infection and bacteria, due to low white blood cell count.

Nurses connected me to a saline drip for hydration. I was severely dehydrated. I did not understand it then, but now recognize the symptoms.

I had to drink more, though in tiny quantities. There is no guarantee that drinking will prevent dehydration, especially during rough patches like chemotherapy and diarrhea. My urine kept going dark, the telltale sign that I must drink more.

After about one week in the hospital, I was sent home to recover some strength before my next lower-dose chemo session started three weeks later. I fell into a dazed state, somehow making it through each day, with not even enough energy to dread the future.

While this drama was going on, my parents decided to sell their Saint-Leonard home of almost 26 years to move closer to their four girls. So they too embarked on their own transition.

The real estate agent was someone I went to high school with. It was awkward having him see me a sickly 94 pounds, even though in high school I hadn't weighed much more than this. But now I was half-bald and wore a kerchief. And I was possibly dying from Stage IIIB stomach cancer.

I was ashamed, and having visitors amplified my discomfort. He never mentioned my gauntness, or my headgear.

I longed to look good. Other women in treatment seemed to manage. Maybe I would have felt a little less sick if I didn't look the part so well. Despite all this wishing, I really didn't have the energy to change things. The real estate agent was kind, but once we had greeted each other, he and my parents went to the dining room and I stayed glued to the couch.

He too had moved from Saint-Leonard to RDP. I ran into him over the years – our children attended the same school and he had run for political office. Whenever we met after my bout with cancer, he always took my hand and told me he was happy to see I was doing well.

Repeated reminders that I was ill came from those around me. No comments were ever made about how I looked – or about my prognosis – during those long months of recuperation. But today, I often hear, "You look really good," "You put on some weight," even "You look tired." I also receive advice, mostly from my family, about taking it easy and not overextending myself.

Recently I met an old friend from high school, and it made me curious about others from our class. It turns out that 10 of my high school class mates are dead. They announced it at our 30th high school reunion, which I didn't attend. Only weeks later, another two class mates died. Former colleagues have also died, among them a good friend who was brutally murdered. These statistics make me appreciate even more the second chance I was given. I hope to live long enough to share my story.

The house my parents were leaving was the home in which my sisters and I each eventually left for marriage. We spent our teenage years in that Saint-Leonard neighbourhood. Susy and I graduated from high school while we lived there, while Mary completed her diploma in our old neighbourhood of Saint-Michel. Lisa was already working at that point.

Saint-Michel, just West of Saint-Leonard, was one of several Montreal towns where many Italians settled after immigrating through Pier 21 in Halifax, Nova Scotia. The mass migration during the second wave of Italians searching for a better life in Canada drove my parents there after becoming independent of their sponsors – my mother's sister. A trail of Italians followed one another from town to town, creating tight-knit communities every place they went.

Parents and children all knew one another in Saint-Michel, as in all the neighbourhoods we lived in. Halloween nights were safe and friendly. The 1970s and early 1980s were a different era. Great memories playing outdoors.

A large park in the center connecting all the roads was the epicenter that attracted the older kids to mingle after school and evenings. My Italian parents were very strict, so my sisters and I usually stayed close to our house. The neighbourhood children shared an elementary and high school.

There were so many Italian immigrant families there, each having an average of three children. I don't remember knowing any other nationality on my street. I do recall having a "Walter" in my kindergarten class at *St. Michael's Elementary School*, but I think one of his parents was Italian.

Today, you seldom see children playing in the front yard – at least not without a parent hovering nearby. Fear is more prevalent today, and I, too, rarely let my daughter stay outside by herself. We are the helicopter generation, always watching anxiously.

The areas I grew up in seem different now that I'm older. The streets are empty. There are few children. Fewer fathers and grandfathers walking the sidewalks and greeting their neighbours. The homes have aged and are not as appealing as the homes in the newer towns in Montreal. We have much to reminisce during drives through the neighbourhoods of Saint-Michel and Saint-Leonard.

At the most recent childhood home in Saint-Leonard, our street was long and led into a slight curve at the other end. My parents knew almost everyone on the street. Susy and I passed by the curve at the end of the street to get to our elementary school. The 10-minute route became less intimidating soon enough. The school sat on the main strip where the local butcher shop was situated, and we often had to stop with my mother to say hello to all the neighbours sitting on their balcony or watering their lawn. I remember doing that walk with my mom year after year until I bought my first car in my mid-20s. We walked the opposite direction to get to public transportation once we started high school and working.

The parents in that neighbourhood are old now, and some have gotten sick and died. The children have all grown and moved away. Other nationalities have also moved in. The homes are no longer dominated by Italians.

Our house was a two-storey semi-detached with a basement. In fact, the street was filled with houses just like ours. As a kid, I had to look for the address on the door to know which house was mine, especially when we first moved there and had to find it after school. Since Susy was eldest, I relied on her to take me home.

The main residence had two levels and included three bedrooms. There were washrooms on each floor, a living room on the main floor, and a very large family room on the lower one. We spent most of our time on the lower floor. I hated living in the basement, but most people who had homes like ours used the upstairs only for sleeping.

We cooked and ate in the basement. The upstairs kitchen was pristine, even the day we left. We kids did our homework on the plastic-covered, now vintage, chrome and lacquer dinner table embellished with cream and brown abstract designs, watched television in the patterned chocolate-and-cream-dizzying-ceramic-covered family room that also housed a bar and wood-burning fireplace. The mirror background behind the bar was used mostly to sneak peeks at our hair and makeup, and needed constant cleaning to keep the glass shelves dust-free.

We were not drinkers, aside from my dad indulging in a glass of homemade wine with dinner, but we always had liquor for guests. All our family gatherings were in the basement, since it was spacious. We could put long tables to accommodate at least 40 people.

Over time, we renovated the basement and exterior. We also remodeled the kitchen. The bar was removed, and the fireplace wall and mantle updated. My father kept the 1975-stamped-at-the-doorstep home in great shape since our move there in 1978.

My father eventually modified our double garage into a real entrance with a brick wall and a door – instead of a push-in door within the garage panel. We played school in the entrance hallway with the other kids many times during the summer. We stayed close to the door so we could catch a breeze.

What is it about kids wanting to play doctor and teacher? Was it curiosity that made us raise our sweater to receive pokes to our stomach? Was it all the hours in school that made us pretend to be disciplinarians, sending each other to the principal's office, or failing someone on a test? We all wanted to be an authority figure. We wanted to grow up.

There were four rental apartments in each of these complexes. It was called a *Five-Plex* – two tenants on the second floor, with their shared entrance from the main balcony that ran the width of the building and an interior stairway leading up to their separate apartments, an independent entrance on the main floor for another tenant, and another for the basement apartment. We also had a lovely entrance, the first door at the top of the balcony stairs, which we only used to pick up mail and take pictures cutting the ribbon on our wedding day. During the hot summer days, I'd exit there to the balcony for sunbathing. We spent so much time in the basement that my father would climb the exterior stairs to sit on the balcony.

It was like living in an apartment building. But each move marked a step-up from our previous residence. And despite being a family of six and often having to share bedrooms, our homes felt comfortable. Life was so simple back then. Those white-brick complexes, with a few beige stones thrown in, and constant upgrades still make me squint when I try to locate my old house on a drive-through.

My sisters and my husband helped my parents search for a home here in RDP. Renovations had to be done when they finally bought a house no more than a five-minute car ride from mine. Only my dad lived there for the first weeks, since my mother was still with me when they made the transfer two months after the end of my treatments in April of 2005. My sisters live in close vicinity to each other, so it's easy to walk between their houses. My house is a half-hour walk away from my sisters'. A car is still more practical to get to my parents' new residence, but Mariano had walked it several times.

So why would my father choose, at such a crucial time for all of us, to move? Moving is one of the most stressful and exhausting things a person can do. Was this his distraction?

When my father decided to sell the Five-Plex while I was in treatment, I suspected he was afraid of losing me. He wanted to be closer to me, even though I was only a 15-minute drive away. This doesn't seem so far, but neither my father nor my mother drive.

Certainly, my father would never admit he chose to move to this new neighbourhood for us, but what was left for him in Saint-Leonard? He made it seem like a normal and logical transition, like all the previous moves.

My father was always canny about the choices he made for family finances. The housing market was ridiculously high in 2005, so he took advantage. And being closer to each other was more practical. It would get more practical still, as my parents aged.

My dad was going to be 81 the summer he sold that building, so maintaining a house and rentals was becoming a big job and demanded more patience than he had. He still bought a big house when he moved closer to us, but he left behind the headache of tenants. Today, my two oldest sisters and their husbands do most, if not all of the work in and around his house, a big property with two kitchens, three bedrooms, a living room, family room, and two bathrooms. Plus ça change ....

Going to the hospital for five consecutive days of treatment became unbearable, especially when the radiation treatments were added.

Radiation being cumulative, I didn't feel the effects right away. Combining chemo with radiation brought me to the hospital again for several days.

Over time, the skin in the center of my torso began to burn – literally. Blackened skin flaked off, revealing reddened skin beneath, too sensitive to touch. By then, I could barely stand up because of all the side effects.

Reducing the chemo dosage a second time still proved to be too much for me. The oncologist's team had to come up with a recipe that wouldn't kill me and would potentially save my life.

My radiation treatments extended through Christmas 2004. I fought for my life instead of enjoying a holiday in my new home. Christmas dinner was usually at my parents' house, but that year we gathered at my house.

While I had always wanted to host a Christmas dinner, the circumstances made this particular occasion bittersweet. Too sick to go outdoors, or dress up to go out for a visit, it turned out to be a wise plan. It was important to me to have that holiday close to my family, and, in a small way, celebrate the completion of our home.

But even being in the same room with others, I wasn't really present. Mostly, they just let me be, not asking anything of me. Too dazed to notice much of anything my frailty dragged itself around the house where groups gathered, until falling again to the couch. Conversations and memories then and in the following months are vague. Being sick took over any possibility of creating any good memory or cherished moment with my two-year-old girl. I can barely remember anything other than being sick.

With the help of my sisters, my mother prepared a superb dinner.

Since my family was there late that night, I hooked up my feeding bag at the usual hour, so it wouldn't have to run the entire next morning. I was forced to walk around with the pole, ticking included.

The liquid entered my intestine one drop at a time. The transparent, narrow, plastic tube that connected the bag to my J-tube sometimes had visible air bubbles. The bubbles never seemed to move, and the level of liquid in the bag never seemed to decrease. Feeding was a tedious process that took about 10 hours to complete. The drops that slowly fell from the bottom of the bag into the top of the tube were the only sign that I was getting any nutrients at all.

At Christmas, my family eats, exchanges gifts, and eats more. We get so full from the antipasti and first plate – usually lasagna or cannelloni – that a break helps us once we get to the long-awaited charcoal-broiled lamb chops that had been marinating for about two days. The younger children are ecstatic about distributing and opening the stacks of gifts they've been eyeing all evening. The overbearing load of gifts were scrunched under and around my tree, bringing disorder to the beautiful Christmas tree my sisters helped me decorate that year. My gifts to the children were cheques that Christmas.

They all played games and cards around midnight. I skipped this part and lay down.

Even though that holiday was agonizing, it established a beautiful new tradition. After that year, Christmas dinner was at my house. My mother was in her mid-60s, and it was time the younger generation took over. I often received help from my family to prepare for special occasions that took place at my house over the following years. I hated that I needed help, but I love hosting.

I was now working with a nutritionist from the hospital. After my follow-ups with the radio-oncologist, I would head over to her office for encouragement and ideas.

She helped me add more calories to my diet than what I had received from the feeding bag. She advised mixing protein powder with my soups, buying meal replacement drinks, and eating high calorie foods. I used the protein powder only a few times in my sweet potato puree, but not in drinks. The sandy texture was disagreeable. The meal replacements tasted like chemicals. They also contained lactose, which my system could no longer tolerate.

My ability to taste had changed. I could taste the chemicals in processed foods now, and they became unappetizing. I had prepared homemade soups and bought fruit in baby-food jars prior to chemo, but once the treatments began, I was too nauseated to eat any of this.

The doctors and nutritionist told me to pack calories before the chemo protocol. My surgeon told me to eat whatever tempted me. But I didn't even recognize hunger until about 18 months following surgery.

They all made it seem so simple, but it was not simple. The cancer patients I now mentor all talk about the challenges with food. They fear trying different foods, and question how much they can eat in one sitting. The doubts come from past experience with vomiting and diarrhea, and painful blockages after meals. There is also the lack of appetite. Recognizing hunger becomes problematic.

I ate what I remembered enjoying prior to surgery. The quantity was my concern. Frequent vomiting and esophageal and intestinal blockages were not helping. I had to learn what and how much was acceptable to my new anatomy. With constant nausea, I soon realized that I had to discover what worked on my own.

Due to the lack of hunger, maintaining or gaining weight was up to me. What I could eat would be learned by trial and error. Over time, my reactions to foods would change. I wasn't gaining any weight, and eating without any visible reward was increasingly exhausting. Three pounds up or down was apparent – that's how tiny I was. I looked to the scale every few days. It was discouraging to see that number go down, but just a two-pound increase would excite me.

Drip coffee reminds me of dirty water, but I developed a taste for espresso – a drink I never liked before. Not many Italians will refuse an espresso. Although the aroma is pleasant, I still don't always like the taste, unless it's sweetened to remove the bitterness.

Now I'm up to a half-espresso from the cup my husband and I share. He was disappointed when we went out on our first date years ago, and I told him I didn't drink coffee. "Now you want to take it away from me," I joke with him. We laugh. He started making a second cup for himself.

My taste buds now crave stronger sensations and flavours, but the patterns of likes and dislikes keep changing, so I'm always learning and adapting. I like caramelized onions and cooked onions in general, whereas previously, I would push them to the side of my plate. Even bitter rapini greens now entertain my palette.

Waking in my own bath of sweat was strange and frustrating. What was happening to my body? During chemotherapy, some nights I would awaken drenched, as though I'd been engulfed in a fire, and the bed soaked by water had put it out. My nightgown clung to my skin. "What the...?" I tried not to wake up my husband who had to work the next day.

Since the operation, I like heavy, layered blankets on top of me in bed. When I don't get hot flashes from the chemo, I get the chills. Between December and April, the house felt cold at 22 degrees Celsius. My husband likes to keep the temperature low – and is constantly checking it. With the loss of fat and the lack of fat absorption, I still felt chilled in layers of sweaters. Other patients also told me they would wake up drenched, and that they are now more sensitive to the cold. I guess it's not unusual.

The ticking of the machine that released the liquid calories through the night didn't bother me, as I was overwhelmed by fatigue. I am a light sleeper by nature and prefer complete darkness in the room, but the chemo and radiation permitted me to tune out sounds and light, and sleep on demand. Often, I'd fall asleep so quickly I didn't have time for prayer. I'd feel bad the next day if I forgot to say it.

It was a miracle when I slept all night. Some chemotherapies, or other medications administered during treatment, are stimulants. Waking in the middle of the night was common for me. I'm not sure if insomnia was caused by treatment or worry, but the sleep disruption made the nights feel grossly longer when I was feeling ill.

If my mother heard me get out of bed, she would come in from her room, the furthest bedroom from mine, to check on me. You could tell she was sleep-deprived, her eyes half-closed, her voice coarse and low. Her mother-love was evident. "What's wrong?" She would whisper in Italian dialect as she stood dazed by my bedside. She was also a light sleeper. She told me years later that she felt helpless all that time that she cared for me.

I couldn't get up and walk around, for fear I would awaken everyone. Reading was out, because it would disturb my husband's rest. My energy was so low that my mind simply drifted. I lay in bed for hours, not knowing what to do, waiting until morning when the rest of the family would wake up. I wanted to be with them, especially with my little girl. I had to wait until my bag was done dripping, however, so I could just disconnect it and head to the washroom for my morning routine. If I couldn't wait it out, I wheeled the pole that held the bag – borrowed from the community health center – right into the washroom a few feet away.

I brushed my teeth first thing. Since my operation, I usually woke up with a film all over my mouth. Lying down caused this, so I began sleeping with a higher pillow. The film was like gelatin, coating my gums and tongue. I avoided speaking because I was disgusted by this mysterious, tasteless jelly. I brushed my teeth and tongue, and spit several times, but the jelly was stubborn. Even when I woke up at five in the morning, which was often, I needed to take care of that jelly.

Occasionally, there would be remnants from after dinner snacks. If I had eaten strawberries, my saliva would be speckled with red. That was always a shock. I thought I was bleeding. Chocolate showed up in the morning too.

I told my surgeon about the film. "Could it be bile?"

He shook his head. "No, you've been reconstructed so that the bile doesn't come up." He sketched one of his diagrams to show the new connections, explaining how the duodenum, I believe it was, prevented the bile from rising. I didn't feel completely comfortable with the explanation, but was assured he was. If it wasn't bile, what was it? I never got the answer.

Other patients of this operation have wondered about the disturbing mouth jelly, and no one I have met so far in my mentoring volunteer work has received a satisfactory explanation. Maybe the doctors just don't know what it is.

Occasionally, I awaken from burning in my esophagus: heartburn, which I did not suffer from before surgery. To this day, lying flat is uncomfortable, so I still use a larger pillow and finally invested in an adjustable bed. If my head is not elevated, I can feel the liquid rising in my esophagus. On occasion, I am still awakened by burning acids reaching my throat, sometimes to the point of vomit. It rushes up so quickly that I have to sit up before it reaches my mouth. Often I have to head to the washroom to rinse my mouth. Clearing my throat just brings the wretched taste up again. Almond milk is the only thing I have found that can calm the burning sensation.

I can eat anything I want, any time of day, but sometimes there are unpleasant consequences. A sweet dessert with lots of cream must be limited to small quantities, or I have to run to the washroom. I am one of the few Italians who has never liked hot spices, so it's easy to stay away from spicy food. French fries and deep-fried foods in general feel too heavy in my belly, so I avoid them. Even small quantities make me feel sick, as though I've overeaten. I cannot drink milk, as lactose intolerance gives me the runs. I use almond milk with cereal.

Liquids can't be drunk with solid food or pain results as the liquid tries to push through the food. Imagine filling a drinking glass with water. If you continue to pour water into it until it passes the rim, it overflows. That is what happens if I eat and drink too much. Space is limited, so getting the most out of my food intake is important. If I ignore the "full" signs, I vomit.

If I eat contaminated food, I know it very quickly. I've also had bad experiences in the better restaurants. The upside is that I relieve myself of toxins quickly, whereas a normal person might feel sick for a couple of days.

My digestion is quicker than that of someone with a stomach. I use this difference to judge restaurants. Certain sushi restaurants that I ate in prior to surgery are now off my list. I am much pickier, the canary in the coal mine. I usually ask for doggy bags when the restaurant food is good, since I usually have trouble finishing a normal portion. Food is richer in restaurants and fills me up quicker; at times, even a few bites cause fullness and sleepiness.

I was in Mary's car with Sabrina and Isabella, heading back from a restaurant. Her husband, Ralph, was driving, and taking us home. I could feel rumbling in my belly. Soon pain began and I sensed a diarrhea attack coming. What do I do?

"Guys, I have to go to the washroom badly."

Mary turned to me with concern. "What's up?"

"Not sure... Maybe it was the food."

They continued with their previous conversation.

My hands pressed against my hot face. I told them I couldn't wait.

"Do you want to stop at my house?" asked Sabrina.

I said no.

"Cherie," Mary said to Ralph. "Try to drive faster."

"I'm driving as fast as I can."

Thankfully, I always did make it safely to a restroom, but there were close calls. No one warned me about the Dumping Syndrome. Normal for me now is loose stools two or three times after I get out of bed. The urge often wakes me up. I feel lower back discomfort until I've emptied my colon. The stools are light-coloured and float. They contain all the nutrients and fat that I ate the day before that didn't get absorbed. This is a disadvantage of not having a stomach. It isn't customary for me to discuss a matter so private, but these details might help another patient to know what might occur.

Anemia forced me to rely on iron supplements, up to three a day at one point. Iron causes constipation. Some days I skipped a dose to avoid bloating in my belly and colon.

In the morning, after visiting the bathroom, I headed to Isabella's room to kiss her sleeping face. She was unfazed by my illness during the post-surgery treatments – the constant vomiting, sleepiness, and sedentary lifestyle. She spent most weekdays with her cousin, Marco, thankfully, so her attention was taken by play or television. But I suspect that even though she doesn't remember it, she feared abandonment. I had left her several times for hospital stays, and she probably feared waking up to a missing mother.

I'd been home with her the entire first year after she was born. She adapted well to spending her days with her grandmother when I returned to work after maternity leave. Hopefully, having us both there during the convalescence helped.

I never worried about Isabella's care. My mother was wonderful. Isabella was well fed, bathed, and surrounded by loved ones. The best part of being home again was that I got to spend each day with both my mother and daughter. I had little energy for interaction, but their proximity meant the world to me.

If my dad spent the night, they were usually downstairs having their coffee and breakfast when I got up. He slept over about three times a week. My mother always made sure he brought food home for the next day. This is how my family has always operated. With practicality and generosity. I realize now what a rare gift it is.

My mom usually tried to get me to eat breakfast, but the nausea often thwarted this. On the rare occasion I could manage, a few bites of toast with butter were a pleasure. I only drank water or juice. Herbal tea became more frequent when plain water began tasting bad.

Once my mother accepted the fact that I was too ill to eat, she stopped forcing. I was still on the overnight calorie bag, so it wasn't fatal. At least my weight was stable, and she soon believed that her daughter was actually eating out of that bag.

The beautiful sound of Isabella calling my name carried through the house so sweetly. I wanted to run up the stairs to hug her. But I could barely get off the couch. My mother ran to her instead, and carried her down the stairs. My heart jumped with joy when I saw the happiness on Isabella's face as she approached me. Isabella's hair, once it finally grew, curled in every direction. Her big dark eyes stared at me with love and wonder. I stared right back with the same.

After Mariano got ready for work, he used to drive my dad back to my parents' house. Some evenings, Mariano would pick him up on his way home from work so he could eat a decent hot dinner with us.

On chemo days, Mariano left work early so I could get to my appointment, usually scheduled at two o'clock. He ate at his desk during lunch. He remembers having to work some evenings. His employer granted him the time he needed for my daily treatments.

With the traffic from the West End, it took him about 45 minutes to get home and then another 40 minutes or so for us to get to the hospital, not including the search for parking. It was costly to park in the hospital lot every day, but he never minded the walk, even in the cold. I was dropped off at the door. He brought his car to the door for me afterwards, while I waited in a wheelchair in the cold lobby.

Mornings and evenings were the busiest time at the house. My sister Mary would drop off her son Marco (then two years old) for his day with Isabella and grandmother. Sabrina, her daughter, attended elementary school. My mother took care of Marco while Mary managed two bank branches.

"How are you feeling today?" Mary would ask, kissing me.

Images come to mind of Mary squatting by the couch where I lounged day after day. Some days I could barely answer; others, I was still in bed when she arrived.

My mother would hand her three or four buttered toasts in a napkin, and she would be off to work until late afternoon. Though I barely remember seeing her come around, she or her husband came every day of the work week to drop off and pick up Marco.

Marco loved my daughter. He and Isabella are nine months apart, and he is always looking out for her, like a brother. He's a teenager now, and once, when we were shopping, he pointed at a piece of clothing and said, "Aunt Patricia, this would be really nice for Isabella."

In my annual Christmas cards to each niece and nephew, I often include a line especially for Marco. "I know you'll always be there for Isabella as you grow up together." The cousins are still close. Hopefully, they will remain so.

On weekends in the period of my treatments, my niece or one of my sisters took my mother grocery shopping. Mariano never did the shopping in our house, except when he needed orange juice, ice cream, or lunch items for the office. I guess we'd unconsciously divided labour on gender lines. If my mother needed something during the week, my sister dropped it off on her way to work.

During those months of treatment, my mother-in-law took the bus from her house in Saint-Michel almost every weekday to help my mom with the children. She reminded me recently that they used to go for walks by the river that is steps away.

Montreal is so cold in the winter, I did not join them. The lowest temperature that year was minus 30 degrees Celsius, with wind chill pushing it down to minus 52. With my drastic weight loss, and now droopy, ill-fitting winter coat, the freezing air tortured me. Rain and melting snow later caused high water levels. I cowered inside.

After breakfast I often told my mother, "I'm going up to take a shower."

"Why don't you leave that today?"

I explained about the night sweats. Even when I could barely stand, I insisted on taking a shower daily. Especially during my treatments, the hot water on my skin felt right, cleansing it of the chemicals that were being forced into my body, and helping me forget for a moment the chills and the sadness.

"Wait, and I will help you," she offered. "*Posso lavare la schiena e i piedi.*" I could wash your back and feet.

But I continued on upstairs without her, pulling my cozy robe close for warmth, struggling to get up the 14 "risers," as my architect called them. I had to raise my legs 15 times to get to the second floor. I felt every step. I avoided going up and down the stairs during the day, except for this morning shower and to turn in for the night. My mother always insisted on getting whatever I needed upstairs because she hated to see me suffer.

I unrobed, trying to avoid the view of my naked, skinny body in the three large bathroom mirrors. The process of covering my feeding tube was a nuisance, but it was the only way to get myself under the soothing water. I had to tape a plastic bag over the gauze. Hot air from the hair dryer after my shower removed any moisture that had collected.

The nurse that came to my house every few days laboured to detach the bloodied cotton gauze from my skin, constantly apologizing for causing pain and discomfort.

I hung the towel over the shower door, and I wouldn't step in until I saw steam. "Ahh!" The heat was too high. I turned it down. I had been told not to wash off the markers penned in for radiation, but that they would undoubtedly fade. Since the stubborn ink never completely disappeared, the technologist could easily redraw the lines, without having to measure again.

One morning it happened. What I had seen in the movies came true. I had never imagined the incredible sadness it would provoke. My hair began to fall out. I was told I would lose about 25 percent of it, but following my first two dreadful treatments, chunks of hair fell out in my hands as I washed it. I lost much more than expected. The balding robbed me of my dignity, my sex appeal, and my hope. I wept. I felt disgusted. I was a young woman, and this particular side-effect from the chemo was a big blow.

I turned off the water and grabbed my towel. Stepping out onto the bath rug, I leaned against the wall by the shower. I couldn't look in the mirrors ahead of me. I wanted my mom to dry me off. Imagine at age 35 becoming dependent once again on your mother. Once I lost most of my hair, I stopped washing it in the shower. I couldn't bear to see bunches of it on the shower floor.

My sisters, Mary or Lisa, insisted on washing what was left in the laundry room sink on the main floor.

Even though they did all the work, I barely had energy for it. I didn't want to face it, so I wore a head-kerchief. The fabric around my head pressed what little hair I had left into my scalp, making it look worse. I kept it covered all the time, so it needed to be cleaned. Looking at myself was intolerable. I could see what the chemo was doing to me. I became afraid to touch my hair, for fear of losing more.

My sister Susy arranged for my hairdresser Giuseppe (also hers) and the esthetician to come to my house. It felt good not having to go out, and avoiding the curious looks. I didn't want anyone to see the ugliness under my kerchief. Giuseppe cut it skillfully, but I still hated it. My face was so tiny and pale. I still kept my head covered because I hate short hair – and bald spots.

Feeling unattractive became the norm during treatment, but I didn't care to fuss with anything. Buying a wig or putting on makeup took energy I did not have. My clothes were all several sizes too big now. My wardrobe became useless, and I had to buy extra-small items for trips to the hospital.

My friends, Annette and Lina R., bought me a black velour hoodie and pant set so I could be warm and travel incognito. I still looked like a famine victim. I learned to layer my clothing, and avoided strapless tops in summer, until 10 years later, when I felt more confident with my body.

Fil, the esthetician waxed my legs on a towel on my bed. My skin had become so sensitive during treatments that the wax felt too hot. We persisted anyway that day. I had become accustomed to waxing myself, but now I didn't dare do it. Fil waxed my legs and then plucked my eyebrows. On the upside, I had lost body hair due to chemotherapy. She refused payment, but I insisted on a really good tip. That was an amazingly sweet gesture on her part. I've told many friends about how she went out of her way for me. Come to think of it, the hairdresser refused payment too. Between the two of them, these two professionals helped me feel like a woman again.

My mother could hear the shower as it turned off, so by the time I walked out in my towel she was there. She could see how drained I was, and she started to dry my legs with another towel. "Ouch! Why are you rubbing so hard?"

She dried my lower legs and feet like she was trying to get rid of dirt. It wasn't funny then, but I am indebted to her.

I don't remember whether it was my mother or me who would remove the fallen hair from the shower, but there was so much, it was traumatizing to see.

I had become the child of my mother again. My own daughter was also now under her care. It was painful to have lost my independence, not only as a woman, but also as a mother. I knew that Isabella would be marked by this important period in her life, and by my enforced absence, but there was no choice in the matter. I had to return to the role of a child because my health didn't permit me being a grown woman and a mother. It was tough to relinquish the reigns of motherhood to someone else, even my beloved and trusted mother.

Relatives and friends came over to visit with me on occasion. They would stay in the dining room with my mother, while I soon headed back to the couch in the family room. I could hear the conversations as I drifted in and out of sleep. No one kissed me during that period of treatments. No one dared get close. My immune system was weak and I could not fight germs. Everyone understood and respected the process.

It was always great for me to see friends and family, and necessary for my mother, who was working non-stop. I should have been entertaining people in the new home, but I stayed at the side, with barely a toehold on life, too weak to join in.

I had no energy to get to know my new neighbours. I didn't feel I looked presentable anyway. Now, after a decade of living here, I sometimes feel like a stranger. The neighbours are kind, but we missed that early bonding period.

Mariano and I live in the first house on the street. We share a fence with the corner house of the road perpendicular to ours where the river (Rivière-des-Prairies) runs. For a decade, we had a stunning view of the water from our kitchen window and backyard. But then the empty lot next to my neighbour's home was sold, and a house was put up immediately. My neighbours are an older Italian couple. They built their house at the same time we did. The man was a landscaper who owned a small enterprise with his son. We asked them to landscape our house. They laid down our stone walk driveway, and all the grass. They also made a cement base for a shed, a stone foundation for a gazebo and dug us a vegetable garden.

When this neighbour learned of my illness, he and his wife came to visit. They were always sweet to me. The woman brought plants she had grown herself. When her vegetables grew through our shared fence, she insisted I keep the string beans hanging on my side. The husband died of cancer only a few years after that, and the wife moved out of the big house into an apartment.

The neighbour directly across from me, also Italian from a home town in Italy close to where my parents grew up, was also generous and kindhearted. She often brought me treats she had made for her family and little gifts for Isabella each holiday. Her frequent check-ins soon turned into a friendship.

An older French gentleman lived in a tiny house to our left. His place reminds me of a cabin in the woods, but it is covered in beige siding. My husband said the house was larger from the inside. My neighbour raised a family of six. He was a cancer patient even before we moved in beside him.

There were many cancer cases around us. A 48-year-old neighbour, who had moved to the street behind us, died of cancer a few years into my recovery. Another woman who lived at the opposite end of our street also died of cancer. Until recently, I was the only survivor. A newer neighbour is now in remission following surgery, and joins me in beating the odds.

Are these cases linked to the neighbourhood environment? It is hard to say. Cancer doesn't occur overnight, and the population is mobile. But it strikes me that this is a small corner to have such a large number of cancer cases.

My husband and I chose this area because it is like living in the country with the amenities of the city only a three-minute drive away. We purchased the land at a steal. The previous owner had combined three lots into one, so our lot is the widest on my street. It's peaceful, with old trees twice the height of the homes, the river nearby, and little traffic, since the street curves and looks like a dead end. Summer is filled with greenery, and the winter forest offers snow-covered branches pretty enough to paint, which Isabella would like to do.

My husband and I visited with the French gentleman in palliative care. I brought him roasted quail in aluminum foil, like I had done once before, when he was healthy and still at home. This time I omitted the wine. Following his death, his daughter had told me how much he had enjoyed that homemade meal. It had been a long time since he had eaten quail, so it was a real treat to have one of his favourite foods again. I wasn't sure it was appropriate to bring the food to the hospital, but I took a gamble, remembering how awful the hospital fare had been during my stay.

When my husband left the room for a few minutes, I asked my neighbour if there was anything I could do or get for him.

"You're very kind... You, of all people, know what's going on in my head." He spoke in French.

I often hear these same words from other patients. People with cancer feel connected. They have all faced a fear of death, pain, and sadness. There is a special comfort they can offer each other, often without words.

I nodded, and we sat in a comfortable silence. We went to his funeral a couple of weeks later. A violin sat atop a stand next to his casket. When I asked about it, his children told me he had been a professional violinist. Now it made sense. In summer, I used to hear music coming from his old, rusted rooftop shed that held a Flintstone pinwheel raised onto its front end. I always thought he was listening to classical music on an old record player. But it was him in there, playing. He used to work with an orchestra here in the city before retirement.

Mariano walked me through the long corridor of the hospital to get to the elevator that led directly to the fourth-floor oncology. When I eventually had to go on my own for follow-ups, I couldn't remember the way.

The department was always bustling with activity, swarmed with patients, caregivers, doctors, and nurses, yet calm out of respect for the sick. The occasional smile on the faces that walked by proved life continued for the well. It would have been nice if someone would liven up the place with more than just the sporadic donor posters and how-to-deal-with-cancer brochures.

It was clear who the patients were – usually the quiet ones or those in line to receive their poison. A few shared their frustration if they waited too long. The visit with the doctor lasted no more than five to seven minutes, with a quick exchange of information about bloodwork, symptoms, and next steps.

Heading quickly to the elevators, I was anxious to return home to get comfortable on the couch.

My treatment appointments often coincided with those of a man who would bring his wife in for similar treatments. At first, we would all walk into the hospital together, and head to our respective chemo or radiation treatment room. Within a few weeks, both our faces had paled, and signs of frailty were visible. Our husbands would haul us in on wheelchairs; we couldn't even walk to the elevator.

For about a month and a half, I received radiation with my chemotherapy. There were 25 sessions of radiation in all – five days a week for five consecutive weeks. I went through the same back door of the hospital for both chemo and radiation, but radiation was in the basement.

Susy had Monday's off. When I had just radiation, she would give Mariano a break by taking me to the hospital herself.

A technologist would be waiting for me down there. Once my gown was on, I headed into the large room. It was very cold, but the whole thing was over in fifteen minutes. As I lay on the cold metal bed, without a sheet to shield me, two women approached. One helped me get comfortable with pillows under my head and knees, so I would stay put; the other checked the markings on my torso, darkening the faded lines with a red marker. They were quite friendly, trying to brighten the experience.

Then they disappeared, and, as I lay still, the two plates that gave off the radiation circled my torso for about five minutes, burning off cancer cells that the surgeon missed or that had grown since the operation. I felt nothing. It's like receiving an X-Ray, very different from chemo. And there was no immediate reaction to treatment. The side effects came later, but the treatment itself was easy.

I close my eyes during X-Rays, an unconscious protection reflex. I did it during these radiation treatments and all the scans. When I reflect what the radiation later did to my skin, it seems childish. There would be no shutting out the pain and suffering.

The skin along my scar went from bright red to dull, dark, and crusty with each session. One day, I was shocked to discover it was black as night, as though someone had torched it. Washing the scorched and flaking skin was impossible. This lasted for months, but with time the colour returned to normal.

Returning home from radiation, I was drained and nauseated. My mother-in-law saw it in my face as soon as I entered. "You're tired, right?"

My mother just took my coat and helped me off with my shoes. I was happy to be home, but too sick to express it. I just wanted to lie down. I washed my hands in the powder room and collapsed on the couch, right next to my bucket.

The children were usually playing and watching *Barney & Friends* at that hour. The purple dinosaur would gather his friends at the end of the show and sing the *I Love You* song. I grew tired of hearing it, but couldn't bear to deprive the kids.

After treatments ended, I couldn't bear that song. It didn't have anything to do with dinosaurs. I associated it with illness. The feeling that comes up is the same one that arises at the sight of the hospital: a brutal reminder of sickness and death, even today.

The week following chemotherapy was the worst. That's when all the little helpers were made available –

painkillers, nausea pills that didn't seem to work, mouth-wash for the sores and swollen gums, hemorrhoid cream for diarrhea, and my bucket for the saliva. I was a slave to the side effects of the treatments as well as the meds.

One morning, during a regular visit by the home nurse, she told me I should go to emergency to have the tube area checked because it was leaking greenish-coloured liquid – a sign of infection. My surgeon was in the hospital that day, and he came to see me in the emergency room. He asked if I wanted to return on Monday to have the tube removed, or if I preferred to do it now. I couldn't tell from his expression if it was a complicated procedure.

I looked at Mariano. Then I asked how it was done. My inquisitive mind wanted to know all before I decided.

"I just take it out."

"What about the hole? Won't it leak?"

"It will close on its own."

I gave him the go ahead. There was a burning sensation in my belly as he pulled out the tube, but it was over in a flash. I had no idea it was so quick and simple.

I was happy to have it out, but now I'd have to get my calories uniquely through my mouth. My weight was very low and nausea was still strong, so eating was a chore. I had to eat six to eight small meals each day. I had no appetite. Eating no longer felt natural – let alone enjoyable.

Discovering what I could eat took months, and once I figured it out, things changed. I had to keep trying foods like meat, nuts, and ice cream, until they no longer disturbed my digestion. Eating frequently made it necessary to vary my diet, since I would get fed up with repetition. Quantities also changed. Ice cream went from none to almost two tablespoons years later, without having the runs.

I had always loved food and enjoyed cooking, but now it became a chore and a central concern. Elaborate recipes were unappealing after cancer, because the preparations exhausted me. I dream of having a chef – even for one year – so I could just eat great food and gain weight.

If I let myself get to the point where my belly growled and a headache came, it was awful, like something is eating me from the inside. I learned the hard way how necessary it was to eat so often throughout the day. The digestion in my body is instant, unless I eat a fatty meal, like beef or Fettucine Alfredo. Certain foods require that I lie down for two hours afterwards, to sleep off the work of digestion. I could feel uncomfortably full one minute, and weak and starving the next. Wherever I go, I now take water and snacks.

For about a year after chemotherapy, I couldn't stand the taste of tap or bottled water. It would have to be boiled and flavoured. So much work! I still sometimes stay away from tap or even bottled water. It tastes as though it's mixed with bile.

The end of my cancer treatments couldn't come fast enough. Susy encouraged, "One more to go!" It seemed like a good thing to her. Theoretically, it should have been for me as well.

Despite the suffering involved in chemotherapy, the end of it can produce internal conflict. You'd think I would be ecstatic about no longer taking poison, enduring endless hospital visits, and throwing up every 10 minutes, not to mention healing the mouth sores, ridding my system of exhaustion and diarrhea and the taste of metal on my tongue. Worse still, the symptoms grew more pronounced with each passing treatment.

Other patients who have completed their treatments have confirmed that, like in my case, the fear of recurrence grows. We have seen our mortality and vulnerability. We know there is no promise that cancer won't return with a vengeance.

For months after the treatments ended, I still experienced side effects, like tingling in my feet and lower
legs. The discomfort stopped me from walking, even
once I got some strength back.

I was consumed by how and what to eat. Each day
I'd realized that all I'd done was prepare food, eat, and lie
down to digest. I was tired all the time and nausea continued to be a daily torture. Housework was out of the
question, so I hired a cleaning lady against Mariano's
wishes.

Scans were scheduled every few months in the
beginning, and eventually, annually. The doctors don't
abandon you just because the treatments end. If cancer
recurs, they want to catch it early.

My surgeon, my chemo-oncologist, and my radio-
oncologist continued to follow me for a few years after
the treatments ended. Suffice it to say, I visited the hospital often. But visiting with the doctors and enduring
treatments are very different.

They poked and prodded at my belly, checked my
neck and underarms for lymph-node swelling, and my
surgeon always had me take a lung X-Ray. Our exchanges were limited, so there was really no reassurance. Only
scans and the occasional gastroscopy gave me comfort.

In my third year of remission, my chemo-
oncologist gave me a thumbs-up. "Usually, with this type
of cancer, it returns within the first two years." He told
me he was discontinuing follow-up, and that I need report
only to the surgeon and radio oncologist from there on in.
It was the best news I had heard since diagnosis.

After five years in remission, I thought it would
be the end of my follow-ups with the remaining doctors.
My radio-oncologist scheduled my last scan. I insisted on

a PET scan. That hospital didn't give those out freely, but she obliged. The PET is more precise and detects cancer cells as small as one centimeter, using radiotracers to detect any problems with organs and tissues. For that reason, it's costly to tax payers. She also booked a partial CT-scan, since it offered better results for the abdomen.

After I received clean results from those tests, the follow-up with my surgeon was the only visit remaining. I was afraid he would drop me too and I would be completely on my own.

But when the day came, he tried to reassure me. "No, I will continue to follow you as long..." He stopped speaking, but I knew what the rest of the sentence was. "As long as you live."

He probably never imagined I'd be here so many years after surgery for advanced cancer. I'm glad I surprised him. "It's over 10 years!" He said during a visit years later.

I don't know where I found the courage, but I shot back. "How many of your patients make it to 10 years?"

The way his eyes widened and his head shook as he kept his lips pursed together said it all.

But the surgeon's glum expression scared me. I thought I had beaten cancer. His lack of optimism at my prospects raised new questions and insecurity.

How much time do I have left? There was no point in asking a doctor. Or anyone. Frankly, death awaits us all. That's our only certainty. The when part is usually a mystery.

The surgeon scheduled annual CT-scans and, every two years or so, I suffer through a gastroscopy.

"C'est à vous *maintenant*." It's up to you now. He held out his hands as if blessing me. "It all depends on how the body reacts to the operation... and if it accepts the treatments."

I never ask for percentages. They can be discouraging. But here is an anecdote to cheer you if you are a cancer survivor. As I write this chapter, it's been 11 years since my operation.

# Chapter 7

# Saying Goodbye

*Why did I get cancer? Who knows. I never smoked and barely drank alcohol. I thought I handled stress pretty well. The culprit might have been heliobacter pylori, a bacteria that causes ulcers and is a risk factor for stomach cancer, according to the Canadian Cancer Society.*

On a hot and sunny June day in 2005, my mother finally moved back to her own house and returned to normal life. She held my frail hand tightly when it was time to go, urging me to be strong.

I am the youngest of her four daughters. I can only imagine how she felt learning her baby had been given a death sentence. Although I don't think she or anyone else in the family knew the details that my husband received about my prognosis, they knew enough to understand I might not survive the surgery and treatments.

Even though I've faced death, I'm still the baby to my family. I feel I've lost my right to that role because of all I have seen, felt, and been through. And yet family continues to shield me from serious matters. I know they want to protect me, and that their intentions are good, but at times they take it too far.

As my mother stood in my doorway clutching my hand, her eyes were full of emotion. Guilt for leaving. Fear of the future. Desire to protect me and take away the pain. "I wish it had been me," she whispered.

My mother was always there for me. She and my father had sacrificed a lot for all their children. We grew up in a strict household, and were taught to be loyal, respectful and independent, work hard, and never take things for granted. We were happy, for the most part, and never spoiled, except with helpings of food.

My mother has taught me a lot about life. Going to the butcher shop with her over the years, I've learned how to choose the best cuts of meat. This wasn't just a shopping lesson. It had wider implications. Her insistence on quality frustrated some butchers, but everyone understood she did it for her family. Although at times her fussiness embarrassed me, I saw again and again how she refused to give her children less than the best on their plates. She earned people's respect for this.

Chamomile tea was always ready when we didn't feel well. The kitchen gave off aromas of a pastry shop. My mother is a fabulous cook, constantly baking cookies, cakes, and bread. The four-layer chocolate and vanilla custard cake for birthdays and other celebrations was her signature piece. It was large enough to feed at least 25. Her Easter bread was sweet and went perfectly with cured sausage. When the grandchildren came around, she baked soft mini buns just to see the smile on their faces.

My mom is the most unselfish woman I know. She put her own health issues on hold to live with me during treatments, at considerable cost, I later learned. I now live with the guilt that her health deteriorated during that time. She had been diagnosed borderline osteoporosis and required calcium supplements and regular follow-ups. She didn't leave my side during my illness and recovery to visit her own doctor or do any tests. And I don't remember her taking any calcium. By the time my ordeal was over and she reassessed her condition, she was well into osteoporosis.

She is always telling us to care for our health. Eat well, see the doctor when we're sick. She doesn't walk the talk. She'll visit a doctor, but her fears get in the way. She's avoided taking a gastroscopy, for instance. I can commiserate. I avoided having a gastroscopy for digestive issues when it was first recommended to me until I no longer had a choice.

Heliobacter pylori ("h. pylori"), bacteria that develops between the stomach and esophagus, before forming an ulcer, is a risk factor for stomach cancer. From that, I experienced bloating and discomfort regularly for a number of years before the cancer diagnosis. I had taken Losec to quell it, but according to my internet research and documentation I received from the *Canadian Cancer Society*, it was likely never fully treated. Perhaps it caused this cancer. As far as I knew, it wasn't in the family genes.

It's so important to pay attention to the body and treat it as soon as something is wrong. I don't regret refusing to take the gastroscopy recommended by my family doctor. I couldn't have known cancer would be my fate. But attending to signs the body is giving is crucial.

After surgery, I was never able to pick up my daughter in my arms again. This was a great loss. I could hug her, but not carry anything heavy, and that meant my child.

Had I known I would get cancer, would I have had a child? Would I even have married? These questions are of little use. I have my life, and I am pretty pleased about the way it turned out.

I've come to terms with the fact that I can't ever be what my mother was for me. I can't be this strong for my own daughter. I cannot do it all, like my mother did. She took care of my home, my daughter, my husband, meals, laundry, cleaning, shopping, and she took care of me, supporting me in my daily struggles with chemotherapy, radiation, and relearning how to eat in the nine months she lived with me.

I no longer have the energy or the strength she summoned to help me. She never complained. She put her own emotions and needs second and gave everything to me. But I knew she was hurting like hell. Parents find the strength to support a child in crisis. I will do the same for my daughter if ever she needs it, to the best of my ability.

When Isabella was three years old, she had an asthma attack, and was in the hospital for three days. I stayed with her. I wouldn't have it any other way and neither would she. She was horrified at the prospect of separation. It was exhausting for me with my weak health, and at one point, I asked one of her nurses to give me a B12 injection that was due. I managed to be Isabella's protector, so I guess the lessons from my mother have lasting power.

My mother had help from my sisters, but the burden was really on her. I don't know how she did it. All I know is how grateful I feel.

Now, when my daughter has an ache or pain, I have to stop myself from fearing the worst. I'm not obsessed with cancer, but I'm certainly watchful when it comes to health. I try to teach Isabella to be resilient and to handle things herself, guiding her to make life decisions that will serve her well if I'm not there. I have also attempted to coach her over the years to stand up for herself, and to respect others and demand respect in return.

When Mariano's brother fell ill with cancer and died, I experienced unbearable sadness and guilt. This was wisdom I didn't care to bear, watching cancer take a beloved family member. I now understood what my own family went through with me.

On the day my mother left my house and my side after the treatments were done, she looked teary. There was so much she wanted to say, so much she still wanted to do for me. Someone had to be strong at that moment.

"Mother, I will be fine."

She couldn't speak. Her sadness got the best of her. Hesitantly, she backed onto the balcony, one step at a time. Then she descended the steps to the driveway. Soon she was out of sight, driven by my sister to her own new home.

I knew there was something I had to do to show my gratitude to my mother. But what gesture could be adequate? Does a mother need a thank you? Yes, she is human. But I know from being a mother myself that the best thanks is seeing your child healthy and happy. I offered her a weekend away together. We would spend time in each other's company away from the sickbed.

But where could I take her? My mom doesn't fly. I would do the driving, and I was still recovering, so the distance had to be reasonable. And apart from the surgery, I had never left my daughter. I asked my mom if there was anything in particular she wanted to do.

*"Voglio solo che tu sei in buona salute."* She just wanted me healthy.

Eventually we decided to book a hotel downtown. Where we were was less important than being together and in decent health.

It was a beautiful weekend. She loved our room. Having a kitchen in the suite excited her. She didn't often travel, so it was a treat for her. I had to convince her that someone else would make the bed. She didn't express joy too openly, yet. Nothing was certain. The past year still hung over us like a cloud, but it was comforting being together for reasons other than being ill. We ate in restaurants, went to the casino, and shopped. A ladies' weekend. Light chat and laughs for two solid days. I hope I offered new memories to offset some of the harder ones.

To this day, I still can't eat or drink much. This is pointless to explain to an Italian woman of a certain generation whose life revolves around food. One of her greatest joys is to feed people she loves. In fact, everywhere we went with her as kids, she had a bag of goodies. Ironically, I'm now the same - albeit for different reasons. Anyone who knows her, knows she makes great meals and desserts, serving them up on demand. It's always been her way of showing love. She still doesn't understand that if I say I can't eat another bite, I just can't. I try explaining that when I'm full I become nauseated and can vomit. But she insists, "Have a tiny bite."

I'm not sure if her fears of losing me prevent her from seeing clearly, or if the belief that food cures all is simply too deeply ingrained for her to change. She continues to worry about my weight, give me heartache that I don't eat her ricotta-filled pastry, or tell me I should eat red meat for my iron-deficiency. Whenever she calls me, she asks if my daughter was well dressed that day or if she ate well. She'll also encourage me to eat more. I often tell her not to worry. I try steering the conversation elsewhere, but she lets up. Food is her love language.

During recovery, I discovered that telling my family I loved them became easier. We certainly love each other, and were always very close; but, like many older-generation-families, *love* was rarely voiced. It didn't come easy for me either, except with my daughter. Not a day goes by that I don't tell her at least once, twice. Well, maybe three times.

Before Isabella, I had practised those words of endearment with my nieces and nephews. With children it comes easily. When I met my husband, and we fell in love, he had not been used to saying *I love you* spontaneously either. I taught him how, even though he'd say it in a joking tone to ease his discomfort. Now that we've been through cancer, even my parents do it.

My mother continues to worry about my health. She tells me not to waste my time doing unnecessary things, especially exercise. I bought running shoes and began walking outdoors. Years into recovery, it felt great to take control of my life again. I had more energy after a while, and felt accomplished. My mother thought I was crazy because I was going to lose more weight. That's part of the reason I avoided exercise during recovery. I just couldn't afford to lose one pound. Now, I try to recover my calories following exercise. My internal voice still tells me *the more you move, the more you'll lose*, but I know building muscle is good for me.

My family worries about my health, and they try not to burden me with their own problems, keeping bad news from me. I've told them over and over to tell me when someone we know falls ill. There have been times when I found out too late. I understand they're trying to shelter me from stress, but with what I've been through, I've learned I can handle a lot.

# Chapter 8

# My Daughter's Gift

*After my operation, I asked my chemo-oncologist about freezing eggs for a second child. In a mechanical voice he said it would take too long and delay treatment. So that was the end of that.*

A year before my diagnosis, I am sitting at my desk at the office, trying to finish a conversation with a client. "I'll have your organization and minute book... ready tomorrow." I take a deep breath, struggling for air. I haven't the slightest idea what could be wrong. I am seven months pregnant and there's a strange tightness in my thorax.

I am carrying pretty high, quite round everywhere. I've gained about 25 to 30 pounds. The pregnancy is normal and all my visits with the gynecologist have gone smoothly. But all of a sudden I'm short of breath now. It's as if I just ran the 100-yard dash. I start to panic.

My gynecologist's assistant tells me I should come in for a consult when she hears my symptoms. The office isn't too far from mine, but since we are downtown, there is traffic and parking could be a nightmare.

I stand in my boss's doorway, teary-eyed, worrying about my baby. I tell him about my breathing. And that the doctor wants to see me. "Would you mind if I left early?"

"No. Go ahead."

"I don't normally take pregnant women off work so early," my doctor said, "but I think in this case it's necessary. I'll give you a note for your boss."

"Should I be concerned?"

"No. Your visits are frequent now, so we'll keep an eye on it. But let me know if it worsens."

In 2002, two months before Isabella was due, I was forced to stop working because of this respiratory issue. The baby was pushing up near the thorax area, making it hard to breathe. This memory came back after my cancer ordeal. The breathing issue might have been caused by tumours restricting the space needed by the baby.

Once Isabella was born, all was forgotten. I cried when I held her the first time. I felt complete. I had never been so happy. So one can imagine how devastating it was to be torn from her life for almost a year. I lost the ability to pick her up when she was just 22 months old.

A few years into recovery, my sister-in-law, Carole, showed me photos of Isabella taken during my illness. My heart skipped a beat.

"I don't remember her at that age." I felt like crying. She and I missed the bonding critical to a toddler. We can't ever get that back.

My sister-in-law was kind enough to give me the pictures, and they still make me sad. Isabella missed out on her mother's touch for too long. I missed out too, on my child's crucial second year of life, and the discoveries she made on her own.

The patients I've mentored over the years asked where I found the strength to get through cancer and cancer treatments. My immediate answer was my daughter. I loved my family and Mariano, but the need to stay alive for my child was stronger.

How hard you fight does not determine the outcome with cancer. Nor will carrying a smile on your face every day kill the cancer cells. You can choose to seek conventional or alternative methods of treatment, but as the surgeon put it, the result depends on your physiology.

Being positive can help you get through some days, but other times, you're too sick for a good outlook. You struggle to get through vomiting, pain, and exhaustion. I hate the phrase "Be positive." All it does is make life easier for others. And sometimes the focus must be oneself.

It is hard to imagine what life would be like for my Isabella if she had lost her mother before she was two. She wouldn't have been the first child to lose a parent, but it's painfully tragic to think I wouldn't have been there to watch over her. Had I not survived, she wouldn't even remember me today, just like she barely recalls my being sick at all.

When I began to recuperate, I often thought about preparing a video for her, so she could have a memory of me. I would also talk to her through important issues of life – health, school and career, relationships, marriage and motherhood, discovering her faith, and self-respect. But I could never bring myself to do it. Just thinking about speaking to a camera about experiences that I wouldn't be sharing with her was too hard to grasp. I didn't want to imagine abandoning her.

I felt absent throughout my treatments. My mother was taking care of Isabella. My daughter and I were side by side, but it was like I wasn't there. We didn't do things together, because I was too tired and sick. Perhaps she learned independence, or perhaps she learned to fear abandonment. I hope it is the former.

Today, I can offer her love, guidance, closeness,

support, and the opportunity to form a bond that felt broken during that crucial year of her life. Optimistically, I would have at least been a good role model – most of the time.

Any lesson must be absorbed for positive reinforcement. As a teenager now, she doesn't always heed my advice unfortunately, but "you'll see when you have your own kids... just like my mom told me."

When I'd be taken to hospital by ambulance, I would get onto the gurney myself. "Mommy's going to see the doctor. The ambulance will get me there faster so I can get home faster. And it's more comfortable for me on the bed. See?"

"Mommy, can I come with you?"

I hated leaving her in a panic, but I had to do what was necessary. I suppose that's fighting cancer.

Throughout my treatments, I'd often go to bed before my toddler daughter. My husband would involve Isabella in tucking me into bed. He would make a game of the liquid food bag he'd hook up to the dispensing machine. He helped her hold the bag in her hands and "shake, shake, shake," then he'd take it from her, careful not to drop the expensive liquid that would feed me throughout the night. After he'd connect the bag to the machine's tube and my J-tube, I'd kiss them goodnight, and fall asleep immediately.

Since that time, I've tried to help Isabella understand my limitations. She used to ask repeatedly why I couldn't play with her.

The whimper was hard to hear, but I was simply too weak to play. Even walking around the room for exercise took all my energy. For the year of my treatment, I watched her grow up at a distance, like a stranger, without the connection we both longed for.

After meals, sleepiness would descend like a curtain and I'd have to rest. I have trouble clearing up the kitchen right away. The rapid metabolism forces me to nap.

One of my brothers-in-law makes jokes about my getting away with not doing the dishes. We laugh about it, but I wonder if he knows that I feel guilty about every-one having to do things for me, even if it's just cleaning up after a meal.

When I host a dinner at my house, I don't eat much. I'm never hungry, and besides, overeating avoids the rigours of digestion in front of guests. It allows the energy to clear up after dinner, so they don't feel the need to. Mariano has to help out.

Timing the preparation is important. Fruit and dessert are prepared in advance. Despite all the work, I love having guests over, so I'm constantly finding ways to handle tasks more efficiently. Meals that don't need much last minute handling provide desperately needed down time before guests arrive. Making the beds, one side at a time, became a habit once using energy had a greater cost. I fold laundry sitting on the couch. Every task must be calculated, in order to preserve calories and energy.

As for my daughter, I find myself trying hard to teach her to be independent early. The probability of my absence in her life has forced me to push her harder than I would have under different circumstances.

I want her to love knowledge, surround herself with good people, and embrace the good and the bad. I show her how to keep order. "You'll want your drawers organized like this, so you can find what you're looking for." I also tell her to ask for what she wants in life, and to stand up for herself. I try to warn her about consumer-ism. When we're shopping and she sees something she likes, she'll say, "I don't want you to buy it, but come and see this." She seems happy just to show it to me. This isn't easy at age five. As she gets older, I show her how to handle household chores and give her responsibilities. She's a quick study.

We may look like a normal mother and daughter, but we are not. We've faced the possibility of early death and loss. It has probably put strain on Isabella but we are bonded. I try to stop myself from forcing her to grow up too soon, but fear speaks loudly.

I have never liked wasting time, and since my illness, that dislike has grown stronger. When I was working, raising Isabella, and taking care of the home, there were projects that needed attending to. I made time for them, even though time was at a premium. Now I realize time is all we have to offer each other. I have stopped living like I'm immortal, like I have all the time in the world. I try to balance responsibilities and desires.

God willing, Isabella learns to accomplish all she sets out to do. I try not to spoil her by letting her have every new item on the market or have her way when it isn't justifiable, but I am confident that I give her my love each day.

I love my Isabella more than my own life, and I want to be able to give her a better world, great health, and genuine happiness. I can't guarantee anything for her. In the end, Isabella has to learn to find her own happiness now that she's older. Hopefully, the lessons Mariano and I are trying to teach her, the guidance we endeavour to offer, and the mistakes we have made on the way will lead to a good and loving life for her.

I've told Isabella and others that having had cancer was a blessing. I would never have had the same appreciation for life and the people who share it with me were it not for that struggle. It was a wake-up call. I was taking life for granted, letting it pass without questioning priorities. What do I want from this life?

On my daughter's third birthday, I threw a party.

My strength was still limited, and I looked like a scarecrow, but I invited about 50 guests. All the families we knew were on the guest list, most of them with young children.

I hired a clown magician for the children. The dove trick made a great impression. Dora, The Explorer, was popular at the time, and one of my daughter's favourite shows, so that was the party theme. The presents she received, especially the Dora kitchen, made her smile. She grew shy when we sang to her and she had to blow out the candles. I have pictures to remind me of that amazing day. She doesn't remember having such an elaborate party, but happily *my* memory was working.

Over the last decade, my priorities have changed. Due to physical limitations and loss of memory and concentration following chemotherapy, I haven't been able to return to work.

Writing has taken its place. It has been my passion since childhood, and I had abandoned it with my office job. Since 2014, I've returned to writing daily. There is a tendency to slack off during the summers, when there are more family events and get-togethers with friends. But I'm always happy to get back to it.

Caring for my only child is the other big priority. In some ways, I feel I've failed at mothering Isabella. She deserves so much, but I've lost so much time with her. Once I was stronger, I did make efforts to be close to her. I began reading to her again every night, and took her with me wherever I went. She made it easy because she was so well behaved. I took pictures with her during every outing. In our photo albums, the gap of the treatment year is evident.

I am so proud of how Isabella handled the trauma. But she says that when people at school discuss cancer, she becomes emotional.

Hopefully she will absorb the good from what our family went through. I want her to know how much strength and inspiration she brought me during the crisis, and I want her to sense and trust the love in our family.

When I was diagnosed in August of 2004, the pedestal of the Statue of Liberty had just been reopened, after having been closed since the September 11, 2001 terrorist attacks, when 2,977 people, excluding the airplane hijackers, lost their lives.

There was an uptick in babies born the following year, these miracle babies signified love in spite of great sadness. My Isabella, though unplanned, also arrived in 2002. In some small way, I have always felt she was *my* miracle. She gave me the courage to conquer each chemo session, every day that I felt worse, and the moments I felt I couldn't handle anymore. She was the miracle that gave me strength during my life-threatening event in 2004.

# Chapter 9

# Testament of My Faith

*I have suffered, it is true. But through the suffering I discovered how blessed I am.*

There are some things I never thought I would have to tell my daughter. She's read my memoir on occasion. I've been quite open with her about everything relating to my illness and its aftermath. She knows that I was lucky to survive. She hears about others we know who weren't so fortunate.

But this chapter is a challenge to write, for I know she'll read it one day. Right now, I think she is too young to understand the contents. Perhaps I won't leave these pages open on my computer until more time has passed.

My menstrual cycle always coincided with chemo. For some women, the cycle stops, but mine never missed a beat. The chemo sessions were every three to four weeks. During recovery, my cycle became increasingly heavy. I bled up to 17 days in a 30-day cycle, causing severe weakness and exhaustion - on top of the symptoms I had from the therapies. My hormones were stirred up by the chemo.

I suffered from anemia for several years and dizziness continued daily. Often, I couldn't stand up due to hemorrhaging. I developed fibroids, and my gynecologist told me I should put off a hysterectomy because of cancer surgery and recovery.

Arriving at a restaurant with friends one evening, I had to rush to the ladies' room because of an excessive blood flow. In the washroom, I made a grim discovery when I checked my sanitary pad: what looked like a bloody placenta, around five inches long. It was dark red and jellied, too big to soak through the cotton layers. I apologize for being so candid, but I was astonished.

I wondered whether it could be a miscarriage. The gynecologist was unable to say, since he hadn't seen it. I searched for images of placentas on the internet, and they matched what I had seen.

Sex was good between Mariano and me. I didn't have much of it during my treatments, but prior to that I had always enjoyed making love. After my surgery, we had to be much more careful. He can't lie on top of me anymore. I still have trouble with any weight on my torso or the faintest touch to my belly. Even a seat belt is uncomfortable if I'm not wearing a coat. You can see the sunken area where my stomach once was. A barium X-Ray shows that my intestines moved to my left side, so there's a vacuum where the stomach used to be.

We had to change the way we made love. I also now get nausea induced by the pressure of penetration. I tire more quickly, so Mariano really has to help.

Only my closest intimates know what I'm about to write here. I hesitate because of the guilt and pain associated with it. I don't want to be judged, but I think I have to speak of it.

A year after my husband's brother died in May of 2008, we attended the commemorative mass in his honour. I had been feeling ill. At the chapel, I was so dizzy my husband had to help me to my seat. I was nauseated and weak. My head felt heavy like a glass ball filled with water and shaken. Before the mass began, the priest graciously agreed that I didn't have to get up during his prayers. Normally, I would not request this, but I was afraid I would pass out.

No one gave a thought to the cause. They knew my health issues. But I had no idea why I was feeling so weak. My iron levels had been low since surgery, but this feeling was different. It swept over me in waves. I could barely get out of bed in the morning, and couldn't get anything done around the house during the day. Cooking was next to impossible, so my husband made a simple supper after work, or picked up something on the road home. I held onto the walls of the house, trying not to fall.

Whatever this was, it lasted a few weeks, worsening with each day. I had to cancel engagements. There was no pain and I was mystified until I realized my breasts were full and hard to the touch, and my menstrual cycle wasn't starting.

I was certain I was pregnant. On Monday morning, I was too dizzy to drive, so I begged Mariano to pick up a pregnancy test from the pharmacy before heading to work. He brought it back to me, then took off because he was late.

Following my diagnosis, Mariano and I knew Isabella would be our only child. Pregnancy was far from our minds as we battled the illness.

I did not wait long before taking the test, maybe only a couple of minutes. I went into the washroom and urinated on the stick, but was too nervous to wait there for a result. But before I could leave the washroom, the stick clearly showed I was pregnant.

I was devastated. With all the chemo and radiation I had been subjected to recently, pregnancy was not good news. And the sickness I'd been feeling seemed like signs that the fetus had been compromised.

When I finally stopped crying, I called my husband on his cell phone. "I'm pregnant," I said, and burst into tears again.

"What?"

"This is why I've been feeling so sick. Something is probably wrong with the baby."

"Why don't you go see the doctor?"

My husband had a hard time trusting urine on a stick would confirm I was carrying his child. When I was pregnant with our daughter he reacted the same way. He didn't want me to mention it to anyone until the doctor confirmed it. But I couldn't wait to spread such great news, so we told our family.

I called my gynecologist's office for an appointment. His secretary mentioned I had to be twelve weeks before I could see him for a pregnancy. I explained that I was at risk because of radiation treatment, not to mention all the chemo, and that I felt extremely ill. She told me to come at the end of the day. I instructed Mariano to meet me there.

I was so frightened and sad. I called my sister Mary.

"I'm with Mommy," she said. We still refer to our mother this way, even though we are mothers ourselves.

"Are you far? Are you almost done?" It was still early in the day, so the odds were not good.

Mary noticed my tone and asked what was wrong.

I told her and cried again. Everyone knew it wouldn't be good for me to bear another child. She told me she'd drop by when she could, but already she had done me a world of good just by listening.

A short while later, my doorbell rang. It was Mary and my mother. I hugged them both, then started to weep.

I did not need emotional support, or so I had thought. Since the diagnosis, support was becoming a habit. Surviving cancer has shown me that reaching out to others is all right. It's so important to feel understood and seen in a time of crisis.

My mother's view on abortion surprised me. She condoned it. She knew a lot about still-borns and miscarriages, because they were so common in her day. Her sister had 12 children, of whom only 6 survived. As much as she loved grandchildren, she wouldn't risk losing her daughter again. I felt deeply loved when she told me this. It was comforting to hear that I was so important to her. Not that I would ever doubt it.

Abortion was not something I had ever envisioned for myself. I wanted children, several of them. I had three siblings and dreamed of making a similar family.

"I'm going to the doctor later today."

"Do you want company?" Mary asked.

I told her Mariano would be there, and she could pick Isabella up from school if we were late. She agreed immediately.

Later that day, my husband sat by my side as I told the doctor how ill I had been lately. He knew my history with cancer and the treatments I had.

"If you were my wife, I would tell you to have an abortion."

I stared at him.

"If you keep it, you'll be very high risk. You'll be followed by many specialists… and nutritionists, to make sure the baby is receiving nourishment, and also to maintain your own health."

"What about all the chemo?"

"We don't know the effects on the fetus. There is a chance the baby will be alright, but we won't know until much later." He cleared his throat. "You'll have to wait until you're seven weeks before the intervention. I can recommend a clinic, if that's what you decide." He explained possible complications if I decided to abort later than seven weeks, or if there were complications during the pregnancy.

I feared serious birth defects. There was no guarantee that my baby would make it. I was unable to nourish myself fully, let alone a new life. I took down the information for the clinic.

The doctor looked at my husband. "This mustn't happen again. It won't be good for Patricia. I recommend you have a vasectomy."

Mariano was taken aback, but we trusted the doctor, who explained the procedure. I wasn't ready yet to have a hysterectomy. "A vasectomy is nothing. It's a simple procedure," he assured us. "I've had it myself."

My husband took the information down for further contemplation.

We had not made up our minds. The doctor was clear. Deep down I knew what I should do, but I hadn't yet committed to it. I had to decide whether to risk a pregnancy, not knowing whether the baby or I would make it. I also had to think of Isabella. I couldn't in all conscious put myself at risk. She was only six years old. If I died, I'd be leaving my husband with two children, of whom one might have serious health issues from radiation and chemical poisoning.

Could I live with a responsibility of aborting a child? Could Isabella ever forgive me if I deprived her of a sibling? Five weeks pregnant, I left the doctor's office with a heavy heart.

I made the appointment with the abortion clinic, uncertain whether I would go.

Two days before the appointment, the nausea and

dizziness were awful. And there was pain in the abdomen. At that point, I understood. I couldn't take this level of nausea, dizziness, fatigue and pain. Intuition told me something was wrong with the baby. I doubted I could carry it to term.

I might have also been pregnant when I had that large jelly discharge. If I waited, my body might expel this fetus naturally.

I finally decided. Thinking of it as a protective health measure, and not a rejection of a baby, helped me through. The fetus's life was at risk, and so was mine.

My husband, mother, and two of my sisters, Mary and Susy, accompanied me to the clinic. My dad and mother-in-law did not know about the pregnancy.

There was a fraught silence, even though my family and I were the only ones in the waiting room. A nurse soon called my name, and my family kissed me and wished me well. I followed the nurse into the procedure room.

Mariano understood the abortion was necessary, and never questioned it. If my family didn't feel right about my decision, they never said a word. They didn't try to influence me one way or the other, and simply showed their love and support.

The room felt like an operating room – brightly lit with lots of machines - a familiar environment in which I now felt comfortable. It was large, clean, and ready for me. The staff were professional and compassionate, from the secretary out front to the presiding doctor.

I lay on the bed, as instructed, and the doctor began with an ultrasound. It was like being in the gynecologist's office – stirrups and all. As she performed each step, she explained what she would be doing. The ultrasound viewer was above me on the right, so I could see what she saw just by tilting my head.

After a few seconds, she looked puzzled, circling my skin with her probe. "I see two sacs," she said finally. She continued investigating. "It seems to be twins." She waited a moment for further reaction from me. "Does this change your decision?"

Thoughts rushed through my mind. I told her it didn't, but in truth, I did not know what to think. Twins would have been an even greater physical challenge and risk. I thought of Isabella, and of my family. I didn't want to die, and I didn't want to bring sick children into the world. I would never forgive myself for that either.

"Are you sure you wish to continue?" the doctor asked.

I don't remember if she asked me whether I wanted to speak with Mariano. Weighing all the possible outcomes, my head insisted it was for the best, so I told her to continue.

She explained the operation. Suction would extract the embryos from the uterus. "Then you'll stay in recovery for a little bit, to be sure there is no excessive bleeding." She said it would not be painful.

Physically, she was right. Emotionally was another story. Within moments, the operation was over. The emptiness and the loss began almost immediately, however, pulling at my heart.

My bed was wheeled into a small recovery area, where four or five other women were already settled on what seemed like stretchers, talking quietly amongst themselves. I was too sad to talk. I asked myself how many abortions were being performed each day. Was life taken so lightly that this was routine? I felt that I would never get over what I had just done.

One woman disappeared to the washroom, and another one packed up and left. Soon we were only three. The young woman to my right said her boyfriend wasn't ready to be a father. I got the sense she was comfortable with her decision, but perhaps she was just acting brave.

My nurse asked me to go to the washroom to check the bleeding. After an hour or so, I too was told I could leave. It was over.

Once in a while, I imagine where they would be in their life. They would be eight years old by 2017, in elementary school, just ahead of one of my great nephews, who entered kindergarten at the same school Isabella attended. I would have certainly sent my other children there too. What a great time they would have had growing up together.

Years later, the memory still haunts me. A mother never forgets. On two occasions, I saw my local priests to ask forgiveness. "Is there any reason it would be pardoned?"

"No, but because of your remorse," the priest assured me as I wept, "God forgives you. You must forgive yourself."

My niece, Claudia, had a miscarriage before her first son, and she had a horrendous time with it. I used my experience to let her know she wasn't alone in her sorrow. We hadn't told her about my abortion, but I felt it was time. I knew she needed someone who could truly sympathize.

She was shocked. "Why didn't you tell me?"

"You were getting married a few weeks later. I didn't want to take away your excitement."

"If I had known…"

"It's alright. Being your maid of honor was an amazing gift to help me cope. And seeing you happy got me through it."

She and I are very close. She always confided in me as she grew into a beautiful woman and mother. I treat all my nieces and nephews like they are my own children – with certain boundaries, of course.

When she asked me to be her maid of honor, I questioned whether she chose me because it could be my last opportunity, or I really was the one she wanted.

She insisted I was the reason, and not the cancer. "You were always there for me. I confided things in you I didn't with anyone else. You knew everything about Frank and me."

That's all I needed to hear.

Intimacy after the abortion reminded me what I had done and what I had lost. The guilt from having sex felt punishing.

"Oh, don't cry."

It's hard for me to admit such vulnerability, but I know there are women out there who understand that making love and children are not distinct.

When I hear people talk about abortion, I fall silent. For many people it's a religious issue, or an intellectual one. For me, it's complicated and emotional and deeply personal. Openness and tolerance are my bywords when it comes to the dread of having to choose between life, death, and abandonment.

My family supported me, but in the end, the decision was mine. It is not an easy act to live with, but I take full responsibility.

A few years later, as my curiosity still lingered, I called the abortion clinic for a copy of the report.

"We only just destroyed the records for that year last week."

Now I will never know whether my emotional scars were for good reason, or if the two sacs were just a broken fetus – if that's possible.

Reminders of what could have been still bring tears to my eyes. My daughter laughs when I become emotional while watching anything on television that involves children.

"Oh... look, Daddy... Mommy's crying."

I'm happy to know she just thinks I'm over emotional, but these sentiments are related to being very ill and losing children I really wanted.

My menstrual cycle continued to worsen. In the two years following the abortion, I had to be rushed to the hospital for excruciating belly pain. I was always dizzy from the anemia, and the bleeding was excessive. The doctor in emergency asked me if I could be pregnant, and I said, "No."

"Are you sure?"

"My husband had a vasectomy."

She shared a smile with her colleague next to her. "Do you know how many vasectomy babies we see?"

Thankfully, the test showed negative for pregnancy. I couldn't go through that again.

The pain came from uteran fibroids. One located near the endometrium was causing the excessive bleeding.

My gynecologist, whom I trusted, checked me every six months. He finally said, "You should seriously think about having the hysterectomy. It will help you."

In May of 2012 I had the hysterectomy. My ovaries were clean, so I still have them. According to his research, my doctor removed the fallopian tubes. That reduced the risk of carcinoma – the type of cancer I had in my stomach.

Accepting that I would not be able to have more children, made the decision to have the surgery easier. Compared to my stomach surgery, this was a breeze.

# Chapter 10

# Struggle for Justice

*So many people die before litigation with insurance companies is over. I fought on behalf of all those struggling with an unregulated system.*

I never thought my life would be like a novel, with such dramatic plots, subplots, twists, and turns. Most of us have drama enough for a book. I struggled with cancer, and after that, battled the health insurer.

My salary was covered automatically for the first two years. In order to start my claim, my employer had to provide salary information, and my surgeon completed several pages about the diagnosis and prognosis, surgery and treatments, as well as recovery time.

During the worst part of my treatments, my salary kept coming monthly, partly through my insurance company and the rest from the government long-term disability pension.

Since I had handled our personal finances prior to cancer, I had to show my husband how to pay our bills online – a new banking method for him. Once in recovery, I sorted and filed piles of papers in disarray. Our house also needed work and attention. Over years, we tackled each project, with Mariano doing most of the handiwork.

Problems with the insurer began after those first two years. The company suddenly refused to continue paying my claim. Some insurance policies put the burden on you to prove you cannot return to work. They felt I was in remission, so there was no reason I couldn't resume my normal life.

I was recovering, with many health issues. The gastrectomy was challenging, and the treatments had lasting effects. Something always needed medical attention. I was getting sick often and recovery was agonizing and took longer. A simple cold lasted two to three weeks longer than usual, and felt more like a flu. Today I still keep an eye out for dangers to a stomach-free body and weakened immune system.

After medical reports and letters were forwarded to the insurance company, I was reinstated almost two years later. My lawyer and I attributed the change to a letter from the initial psychiatric/psychology team.

What disturbed me most was that my physical limitations had no bearing on the decision. I couldn't understand why fear of death took precedence over my inability to function normally due to digestive issues. How was it that the need for constant breaks, states of chronic fatigue, and memory loss weren't considered reasons to prevent me from holding a job?

I challenged the reasoning with my lawyer, but we decided to leave it alone. I insisted, however, that she include physical limitations in all future correspondence with the insurer.

About two years following reinstatement, the insurer stopped covering my salary again. The government disability pension was never interrupted. An insurance agent called me and advised that, "Since there is no proof of your inability to work, we are no longer paying you."

I told her I was grossly underweight at about 104 pounds, and struggling to keep that weight on. I became so frustrated by the agent's insensitivity, I hung up.

From then on, all documents sent by my doctors were ignored.

The September 2008 financial crisis saw a drop of almost fifty percent in the stock value of this Canadian insurance company. It declared huge losses due to its exposure to segregated funds. Financial markets around the world were negatively affected, almost bankrupting this well-known insurer. The business sector reacted with caution, and effects rippled into our homes.

In my opinion, this Canadian insurance company, having huge investments in the United States, was scrambling to recoup its losses. I would have done the same. Insurance agents were likely told to curb spending as much as possible, which unfortunately, may have affected my medical claim.

Insurers often try to push claimants into finding lower-paying jobs with a new employer. When my insurer acknowledged that I was unable to fulfill my own job requirements, it provided me with a list of jobs for which I was overqualified. I did not think I'd be able to fulfill those job requirements either given my health, but the insurer believed I could.

I tried explaining to the agent that losing my stomach was a permanent change that had completely altered my life. They said that my complaints were "subjective, and we need to see test results proving your inability to return to work."

I sent the insurer a copy of a study that recognized that chemotherapy causes chronic fatigue that lasts for years. There were no available studies on the effects of eating without a stomach.

My surgeon told me some patients return to work after a few months, but he hadn't taken the incapacitating chemo and radiation treatments into account. No one knew for sure that I would make it through surgery, so full protocol was not considered part of the recovery period.

I occasionally had intestinal cramping. Excruciating and debilitating pain following the gastrectomy. Certain foods forced me to lie down.

Patients I've mentored described the same type of pain, and having to get their abdomen pumped to remove the blockage. My blockage was probably caused by a steak I shared with my daughter at lunch that day. I didn't touch red meat again for many years.

Prior to cancer, finding a job was easy. But who would hire me now knowing I would have to eat and take time to digest every two hours? I was not about to lie to get hired and then have to admit all my health problems. In most health claims, the doctors hired by the insurance companies will find you able to return to work sooner rather than later. To top it off, the insurance company had no incentive to keep paying my claim, since my employer had taken his business elsewhere soon after my surgery.

I refused to give up fighting the insurer because of the injustice. It consistently ignored the physical limitations caused by the surgery and treatments, and disregarded my doctors' assertions that work would be detrimental to my health.

The doctor hired by the insurer, a retired general practitioner, "read" my file and said he didn't agree with my oncologist, psychiatric team, and other doctors who had been following me for years. He never met or spoke with me. He never examined me. He probably didn't even know the details of my condition. Most people give up fighting an insurer because they think they'll never beat a powerful corporation.

Reputable medical internet sites suggested that most people who had suffered from stomach cancer and had a partial or total gastrectomy didn't survive long. There is little information available for those of us who have survived over five years.

Since we don't know the long-term effects of a gastrectomy, health concerns can't be predicted. My age may mislead doctors. All I can do is pay attention to my body, and bring up concerns with my specialists. I have a lot to say about living after a gastrectomy. Doctors may not be fully aware of what's going on in an anatomy like mine. They know which tests and solutions are necessary, but not what happens in the long term.

I instigated court proceedings against the insurer. In front of the judge during a settlement conference, their lawyer denied documents that had been previously pre-sented, as well as recent letters from my doctors clearly stating I was still unable to return to work.

My employer always kept the door open for me so I could return whenever I was ready. But years later, I'm still at home. I miss the office and the paperwork, alt-hough I'm afraid of a level of responsibility and stress that I may no longer be able to handle due to concentra-tion and memory issues. Learning is also a challenge.

My employer represented me pro bono against the insurance company. It became a fight about principle. I wanted to stand for those who couldn't afford to fight in court. I couldn't afford it either.

We eventually settled out of court. The settlement should have been higher, since I'm still unable to work, but I was anxious to stop fighting, and my boss, Howard, felt the same.

If you are privileged enough to have disability insurance and have the unfortunate experience of needing to use it, fight any injustice as best you can. Lawyers are expensive, so try all other resources in your area, such as Legal Aid - but to be eligible you have to be without means. Struggling is not enough. Make deals with those who can help you, but be sure you can fulfill your end of the bargain.

Insurers don't like people who fight them. Don't take it personally. You are a number in their book, nothing more. They are trained to make you feel there is no hope, and that you are trying to scam the system. Fight for what is right.

# Chapter 11

# Volunteering

*"...Patricia has been my mother's lifeline...
What I have realized is that no matter how
supportive the rest of the family is to the patient, it doesn't begin to compare to the support offered by someone who's actually been
in the patient's shoes."*
Quote from a letter sent by a family member
of a cancer patient. Reprinted with permission from the Hope & Cope Newsletter, Fall
2007, page 5.

After surgery, and before my radiation and
chemotherapy began, I was put in contact
with a volunteer from Hope & Cope. Volunteer-based,
Hope & Cope, a well-known and beloved association
located in the Montreal Jewish General Hospital, offers
support to cancer patients and their families to help with
diagnosis, treatment, psychosocial needs, and bereave-
ment.

I contacted a volunteer a couple of times who had
experienced the same cancer and treatments that I had.
He was about a year ahead of me in the medical process
and some years older. Optimism grew after speaking with

another person who had made it through, against the odds.

Unfortunately, once treatment began, I was too ill to phone him. Speaking brought on nausea when I was undergoing chemotherapy. I gagged if I spoke more than a few sentences.

Nausea still affects me, albeit less often than in the first eight years following treatment. It rises up when I speak for a lengthy period, become stressed, or overeat.

A year or two into recovery, I contacted the same man once or twice more to see how he was doing. I was always afraid to call and find out he had died, but each time we made contact, he was well.

When I asked him about maintaining a healthy weight, he told me his wife took very good care of him, preparing "lots of meat and potatoes." I could tell he had a smile on his face. He had put on 20 pounds since his lowest weight. What I would give to put on 20 pounds. He taught me that gaining weight was possible. Our conversations helped me heal more than my body.

As I struggled to rebuild my life after cancer, I realized my fear would never completely leave me. Sharing intimate feelings with a fellow survivor, helped calm the fear.

I decided to offer this same gift to fellow patients. It is important to know it is normal to be afraid. Patients need to feel seen, and have the freedom to talk about what they're going through.

Many of my emotions during treatment went underground because I was so sick. I couldn't face the fear of death or how to live after cancer. One time, sadness welled up in me quite strongly.

I was sitting in my usual spot on the couch in the family room. My mother and mother-in-law were chatting around the granite-top island in the kitchen. It was after lunch, and the children were having their nap, snuggling on another couch with blankets and pillows. They each also had a stuffed dog my mother had bought them when they were born. Marco's was blue and Isabella's pink, otherwise they were identical.

Suddenly, I burst into tears. I turned my head away from the kitchen, hoping my mother wouldn't hear me, but she asked immediately what was wrong. "Nothing," I said. I wasn't completely sure.

"So why are you crying?"

"I just feel skinny and ugly with this handkerchief on my head." But it was more than that. It was the kids, lying so near me, but out of my reach. My mother standing nearby, but in another realm from where I lay. I felt so alone. There was support all around me. The nurses and doctors all commended me on my family. And yet I felt no connection.

I had a similar meltdown in my dining room one evening, soon after my diagnosis. My husband and I were finishing dinner. Isabella had already eaten and was playing in the living room, oblivious to the horror that had befallen our family. Mariano and I were talking about gastric cancer.

He reminded me of a time, at the beginning of our relationship, that he had taken me to a park one Saturday. On top of a small, rolling hill, we lay on a blanket on the grass. It was green and tranquil, with a view of Old Montreal across the river.

Mariano and I were getting to know one other. He was 35 and I was 29. As day turned to evening, I got hungry and told him we should get something to eat.

"Soon," he said. "Let's relax a little longer."

So much time went by before I could get him out of that park that my stomach cramped. I didn't tell him right away. When we finally headed to a restaurant, the pain was so great I had trouble eating.

Mariano also admitted in recent years that from time to time back then, he could taste or smell something odd during a kiss. "Like raw meat or blood." That shocked me. No one likes bad breath.

While talking with Mariano that night, I suddenly felt the gravity of my deteriorating health. This wasn't a fever or a sprained ankle. It was life or death. Tears started, so I rushed out of the room. I didn't want Isabella to see me cry.

Heading toward the family room, I found myself looking for support from the wall where that three-picture vertical frame now hangs. I broke into a desperate cry, unmasking the fear that finally told me I could be dying.

Mariano walked over.

"I don't want to die."

My daughter must have noticed we were gone in that big house she initially found intimidating – a house not big enough to silence the sadness. She found us soon enough, and wrapped her tiny arms around my leg, sensing something was wrong. Resting my hand on her head was about all I could manage, as I tried to hold back my emotions. Finally, I whispered, "Mommy loves you."

My husband didn't say a word. He stood close, but I don't remember a touch, maybe just his hand to mine. I could see his emotions, held in check behind closed lips and flushed cheeks.

In February of 2006, 10 months after my treatments, I called Hope & Cope to volunteer. The Survivorship Program Coordinator, Hinda, told me it was protocol to wait one year following the completion of treatment. This ensures a stronger mental, emotional, and physical capacity to offer strength to others.

She emailed a profile form to complete with personal details, diagnosis, and treatment information. Another application went further into my experience with cancer, requesting details about how I coped and what I could offer others. We also spoke about my interests in volunteering and what services I could offer. Peer mentoring – telephone communication with patients or family members – sounded great because I wouldn't have to leave the house and it was the most time efficient type of work. She liked what she heard and read from the forms I submitted, so she decided I was ready. I was excited to get started, even though I wasn't sure if I would do well.

Aside from my aunt, who had died 18 years earlier when I was in my early 20s, I had never been close to someone with cancer. After training sessions with Hope & Cope and initial interactions with patients, I knew I had found a calling.

Helping cancer patients involves sharing my own experience, listening, and just being available. Most patients and caregivers are scared to death about the future, the suffering, and the loss. Volunteers offer connection, hope, and someone to lean on.

There were periods when I had more than five patients at a time, so I kept notes of each conversation. I didn't want to forget what stage each was at or mix up their stories. Soon the personal connections made it easy to keep up with where they were in treatment and determine the frequency I should be calling.

As patients, we need acknowledgment of our fears and our suffering, not judgement. Isolation diminishes as we find confidence in sharing our deepest, but common, feelings about death.

I update the files periodically with details of major issues and developments in people's lives, including death. If I got to know family members, I sent a sympathy card.

It helps me to know I am helping these families in some small way. Facing my own death has changed me. So has knowing that my remaining time might be brief. Only one who's been there can understand these particular fears.

Serious illness affects all those around us, so I sometimes stay in contact with a family member after a patient dies. Everyone reacts in their own way to illness, and it can vary from denial to anger.

Volunteering has helped me to feel and articulate my own hard emotions. So I cannot go on without thanking all the patients and families I've had the privilege of speaking with over the years. They gave me a sense of security in my own journey. Their example in reaching out for help, especially when the outcome is grim, is inspiring. No one should have to go through cancer treatments alone.

My work as a peer mentor for stomach cancer patients has been one of the great gifts of living after cancer. Survivors are few, and I'm the only volunteer of my kind on staff. As soon as a patient or caregiver requests assistance, I am called. Details known about the patient's diagnosis are provided. It is up to me to contact them immediately and regularly.

In every one of my cases, the relationship has been a success. Hope & Cope doesn't impose its services. People who contact us are highly motivated. The foundation also offers wellness classes, events, and a place outside the hospital environment for patients to share and relax with others. A home next door to the hospital was bought and renovated, and now accommodates various free classes and activities. These services are available to patients in treatment at other hospitals as well.

One patient who had refused treatment suddenly went missing after six weeks of conversation. I could no longer reach her by phone. Through Hope & Cope, I learned she was in hospital. We spoke two or three more times and then she died, days later.

Another man, with whom I was in contact with for three and a half years, ended our conversations when his cancer returned after remission. He told me that I couldn't understand the hopelessness of receiving a second death sentence. I gave him his space. But after a few days, he contacted Hope & Cope wishing to speak with me again. He died shortly after.

I mentored a lovely woman over the phone for just over a year, and when she moved to palliative care, she wanted to meet me. I visited her at the hospital, and then attended her funeral to support her family.

Recently, an older gentleman who clearly did not wish to share his fears, kept asking me to call and not forget him. I learned that just being there with small talk can be enough.

My contact with many of the patients stretched for months and years. Sadly, most have died, except a French-speaking man I was paired with over a decade following his total gastrectomy.

I cut contact with some patients who were in stable remission, in order to make room for the newly diagnosed. One of my "graduates" got sick again and died recently. Her daughter called Hope & Cope to let me know.

A cancer patient with a daughter Isabella's age shared her worries with me. We were both troubled about abandoning our children, and worried that we would not have enough time to teach our daughters resiliency.

Like many patients, this woman comforted me, lessening the loneliness and fear that death could be near, even if this often went unspoken.

The people I talked with were grateful. As a peer mentor, I speak to patients on the telephone. Only occasionally do we meet in person. My weakened immune system doesn't allow me to visit hospitals and risk catching bacteria like C-Difficile, an on-going problem in many hospitals. Some volunteers attend to patients in the hospital.

Another reason I prefer the telephone is that I am

shy. My best exchanges with patients have been on the phone. On rare occasions I met them face-to-face. Part of the reason I keep that distance is to avoid emotional stress. I am a volunteer, not a member of their intimate circle. Friendships do form, but it's a relationship with enough distance to protect us both.

A passion was awakened through these interactions, a passion for helping people live, not simply survive a hopeless diagnosis.

Offering support is simple. The main requisite is to drop judgement, whether or not we are cancer survivors. It's impossible to know the other's pain, tolerance, or fate.

We all have something special to offer others, whether that other is a friend, a relative, or a stranger fighting for his life. It is often easier to share our suffering with a stranger, so we don't burden loved ones. Some patients don't even have family or close friends they can turn to for support. A simple "let me help you," goes a long way.

Don't wait for a person in need to call for help. He or she may never do so. Just show up and offer. When I was desperately ill, this was how I discovered genuine friendship.

Sabrina, Mary's daughter, participated in a Terry Fox Run with her school in 2008. Imagine how touched I was and the awful memories that filled my head anew when she handed me a small poster that hung from her chest during the run. It read, "I'm running for my Aunt Patricia." I still have it, and remember all the colours she used to write the words. It was a beautiful gesture on the part of my then 10-year-old niece, but painful to think how traumatic the event may have been for her as well.

Some people ask how I can bear watching people die. Why would I want to expose myself to this, when I myself have been mortally sick? The secret behind volunteering is that you receive far more than you give. Volunteering gives my life meaning. The feedback and appreciation bring serenity and a sense of personal fulfillment.

It is daunting knowing you're on your deathbed. It is horrific not having anyone there to help you through it. Most people want to feel love more than ever during their final moments – to share emotions they would never otherwise reveal. None of us wants to leave this Earth alone.

I am appreciative to have a big family that is always there with me, even though we don't necessarily talk about our emotions.

Now that I know about Hope and Cope, I wish I had sought more of this kind of care during my own battle with cancer. I was too ill and tired to understand my emotional needs and take advantage of the services offered.

Cancer support groups help deal with symptoms. You may even make new friends.

My work as a peer mentor is so rewarding that I intend to continue … for life!

# Chapter 12

# When All is Said and Done

*People move on. We all should.*

As cancer patients, we transform. Returning to a normal life may no longer be possible. It's often a challenge to accept the new reality, and judgement from others doesn't help. I have daily reminders of physical and emotional losses. Fear of illness and death can be strong.

After my diagnosis with cancer, planning events more than a few weeks in advance felt counterproductive. Organizing parties, fundraisers, or even a vacation seemed pointless. I visualized being hospitalized, with tests showing the cancer had returned. Planning would have been a waste of time, energy, and money, when I could have just enjoyed each day with my family.

My body spoke up louder than ever before, following the gastrectomy, telling me what it couldn't handle. I often put off a walk or hosting a dinner party for lack of energy. When someone suggested a trip or outing months in advance, I used to cringe. As far as I was concerned, each day was a gift. For many years, I could not see beyond that.

Eventually I accepted that life affects the body's energy. And fears must be fought. Living solely in the present sounds great, but it's impractical. Once I let the fear of illness and death fall away, I could see myself more clearly, with my strengths as well as weaknesses. I was alive. I was in remission. Perhaps not forever, but I realized that so much time went by since my remission began, that maybe, just maybe, I'd be ok. Dare I speak this out loud?

Learning to live this new life means giving priority to eating and resting. Now that I am comfortable with the changes, I can start building a life to respect them.

My priorities are to be a good person, mother, and writer. I also want to share my accomplishments with others. While respecting my health, I am also moving toward these other objectives, and to finding fulfilment in this endeavour.

My father is in his 90s now, and he sees his end approaching. When he complains about ailments, I remind him of his long life. There's much to be grateful for, despite the aches and pains. Knowing you've seen your children grow, held your grandchildren in your arms, loved, and created lasting memories for generations can ease the suffering.

It's hard not being able to walk, feeling lonely, or living with daily medical issues. It's also really hard to face death. There is no easy way through. All we can do is realize how human this experience is, and try to be there for our own anguish and for that of others.

Hard experience can be used for good. Maybe that's the purpose of suffering – to humble us and help us understand this truth. Being with others in their need offers them the opportunity to share their wisdom and see their own strength.

In the spring of 2009, doors opened for me. I started a handmade-jewelry business. It was the beginning of my entrepreneurial career and another way to contribute to cancer awareness. It also helped me get back into the work environment that I missed so much. It wasn't stressful, and there was a creative aspect. For three years, I donated part of the profits to the Montreal Thoracic Surgery Research Foundation, a cancer research group my surgeon co-founded in 2004 – the year I was diagnosed. I wanted the money to go to stomach cancer research, but the foundation concentrates mostly on the lungs; including, transplants. Regardless, it was a small gesture to the surgeon and hospital that helped me live.

The business was great, but I needed even more of a creative outlet. Soon after the litigation with the insurance company ended in February of 2014, I decided to write a cancer memoir.

I've been writing since my adolescence. I completed a novel in my early teens. I remember the joy and satisfaction as I sat on my bed and typed that novel's last line. I also wrote poetry, articles, short stories, and some non-fiction memoir pieces. When I was diagnosed in 2004, my creativity disappeared for almost nine years in the fog that muddled my brain. I wondered if I would ever be myself again.

My psychologist was happy about my memoir idea. She thought it would be therapeutic to get my feelings on paper. She is right.

Returning emotionally, spiritually, and physically from my protective state ushered that voice to scream... *It's time to write again.*

Telling this story is important for me. Apart from the peace and awareness it brings me, it might be of help and comfort to others.

Writing stories takes time. It can exhaust you, and

isolate you. It also has many rewards. When the urge drives me to write, it's hard to stop. Time passes quickly, like the short summers here in Montreal. I take my laptop to the balcony in the backyard. Writing releases adrenaline. And I've been soaking up Vitamin D out there. I'm eager for that rush of trying to write faster than I can think.

Memories pop up constantly. If I didn't write them down, they would vanish. Pieces of paper still sit on my desk, my night stand, or inside my purse. Little treasures I have found to insert in the story. Cell phones are great to record emerging memories. The more I write and read, the more inspired I become. The jewelry business was put aside, mostly because the intricacies of making jewelry was hard on my worsening eye sight.

After a few chapters of the memoir were written, I re-enrolled in an online novel writing program I'd started 20 years earlier. The *QC Career School* based in Ontario reinstated me for just 80 dollars to cover the new materials. I entered the three-year program in May of 2014. I tried to work on both fiction and the memoir simultaneously, but it was problematic.

I began submitting each chapter to the tutor for review, and heeding her advice. It took less than 18 months to complete my first draft. Thinking deeply about my recent past helped clear my mind and put things into perspective. Whether I will be able to sell the memoir is a mystery, but writing it has been transformative. Regardless of its fate, writing will always be a part of who I am – whether I am good at it or not.

It would be so nice to say I have a published book, but the process is slow. I'm not there yet. I'm still working. I am happier with the result than I expected, and relieved by encouragement from my friends and blog readers.

It has taken three years to write. Further editing will be entrusted to a local professional whom I can have a relationship with going forward. The process has been one big learning curve.

In 2014, I also completed 10 years in remission. My niece, Claudia, told me to have a party, but my sister Susy had just announced she was divorcing her husband after 25 years of marriage, and no one in our family was feeling festive. The 10th year of remission did feel really special, however, and I was full of hope for the future.

I wanted to commemorate the anniversary in some way. Susy's separation gave me a sense of calm and perspective. The jab helped flush the demons that kept me from living. I was here and well now, in sound body and mind. My focus shifted from my own fears to her. I could support her through her life change.

Realizing that others in my life needed help freed me from concentrating so hard on my own situation. I stopped seeing my psychologist. I did not want to spend the rest of my days focused on a disease. Volunteer work had taught me that fear shrinks when you speak about it. This work also helped shift my focus to helping others deal with their fears of suffering and death.

Writing this memoir fits in with this vision. Hopefully the book can offer comfort to people with life-threatening illnesses, their caregivers, or even those who fear them.

It took me almost a decade to understand the hope in life after cancer. If we let fear of death or recurrence dominate, life after cancer can become a hell. The fear never leaves, but it does diminish, or at least it can be put in perspective. I do know that I must live my life to the fullest. That is what suffering teaches.

Surviving cancer has brought me many things. I learned to speak out. I'm writing again. My faith in God is stronger, and I talk about faith more openly. My perceptivity has grown. The openness that I wouldn't allow myself previously has forged strong relationships.

People tell me that they don't speak of cancer or ask me questions about my health because they don't want me to feel uncomfortable. But I actually welcome the subject. Talking about it has healed me, and might help heal others. The fear is not only in me, I have come to realize. Sometimes people protect themselves from any mention of sickness or death.

Anxiety occasionally sweeps over me like a riptide. My chest tightens, and butterflies race in my abdomen. Sometimes I take a stiff drink. For me, "stiff" is light alcohol content. And I only take a couple of sips. Usually that's enough for calm to return. My body reacts quickly and not always pleasantly to alcohol, so I doubt I'll ever become dependent. But this danger is something for survivors to watch for.

My journey of discovering who I am, and learning to embrace my life after cancer is daunting. Finding true happiness and fulfillment are as large a part to my recovery as is learning how to live without a stomach and the capacities I once enjoyed.

The knowledge that time is limited creates pressure to complete goals. Others are affected by my choices, however, so I've had to look hard at what I value. My husband is less than happy that I spend all my time writing a book that may never sell (though he understands the obligation to the craft), but this is truly important to me right now.

Though some people return to living the way they did prior to a trauma, I did not. I now want more out of life, more quality, rewarding relationships, rewarding activity, and putting my creativity to good use. When I go, I want to be remembered as good-hearted and loving, a mother who deeply loved her daughter and gave her what she could, a wife who cared, a daughter who honoured her parents, a sister that you could turn to, a friend who made you feel welcome, and a writer who touched others. After being on my deathbed, I'm just starting to live.

The Christmas party I organized each year for Howard's law office still went on in 2004, when I was hospitalized for serious neutropenia following my first chemo treatment. Our entertainment lawyer, Stephen, whom I've known since the early days at the firm, had a picture made with the staff holding letter cards that spelled out "We miss you Patricia." It was sent to me with a beautiful card filled with warm wishes.

Even working a few hours a week will cause exhaustion and, not having enough time to eat all my meals would certainly bring malnourishment, despite the years that have passed. My stomach hasn't regrown, so I have the same issues I had a decade ago.

An MRI of the brain showed chemo residue in the white neurons – if that's how you explain it. "I see this in diabetics," the neurologist said – something I am not. This was the reason I was having so much trouble concentrating and remembering. She advised my insurer. It's comforting to know there's a medical explanation for my confusion and lack of coherence.

# Chapter 13

# Renewed Strength

*"...My favourite black lace dress hangs in my closet. If anything happens to me, I would like to be buried in it."*

Two friends and I took a trip to Las Vegas in June of 2016, once our daughters finished elementary school. As I exited the large washroom in our hotel room with my bathing suit and cover up, I warned the girls about my belly scars. They were friends from after my illness, mothers of Isabella's school friends. Although they knew about the cancer, they had never seen any evidence.

"Let's get this out of the way," I said. "I don't want you to be shocked at the pool."

They told me it was okay. They didn't need a preview.

When I visit doctors for me or for Isabella, and must reveal my health history, shock registers on the doctors faces when I mention my cancer. Stomach cancer at such a young age surprises everybody, but my surgeon tells me that more and more, stomach cancer affects the younger generation.

Stomach cancer is widespread, even though you

hear less about it than breast or prostate or colon. Asia had the highest incidence of stomach cancer in 2012, according to *World Cancer Research Fund International.*

Stomach cancer has a low rate of survival. I am grateful for having overcome the odds, and don't pay much attention to statistics anymore. Friends and some doctors are curious about symptoms, and how I manage without a stomach.

"You are my miracle patient, having beaten all statistics and made liars out of us doctors," my surgeon pronounced.

"I am thankful every day for what you did for me. You were the only one that left out the negativity and treated me like I had a chance of surviving this."

One of my doctors who seldom sees cancer patients asked me how I dealt with it, and what one would say to someone who has cancer.

There is no right answer. But small gestures can have big impacts, so offer the help that you can. Being available, whether being present for a treatment or for emotional support, is the most important. No one should be alone during such a trying time. Join them for a walk, accompany them to appointments, bring them takeout or something they like eating, walk their dog, or just spend some time with them. Some may not feel well enough all the time, but keep trying. Can you offer to do chores for them, pick up their medication, or take them places they need to go?

"I'd like to come to one of your treatments," my boss, Howard, said one day. And he did. His concern didn't stop after the hospital visit following my surgery. He often called to see how I was doing. If I was too ill, he would engage my mother in light conversation, allowing her to use her broken English. My mother raved about his thoughtfulness.

The day Howard joined me in my chemo session was funny. Mariano went for rice pudding at the cafeteria and a walk, so Howard and I could catch up.

It was an especially cold winter day, but that never stopped Mariano from being outdoors. Friends are amazed that he will walk for hours in bitter cold, with his layered thermal clothing.

When I'm receiving the chemo treatment, I'm consumed by images of my cells under attack, like ants in an ant trap. I am disgusted as I watch the liquid being pushed into my tiny veins.

The nurses came periodically to check on me or to change the medication from anti-nausea remedies, including Benadryl, then to another, then a rinse, then the chemo, and finally another rinse. Each patient in the long, narrow room had his or her little space; and, aside from the occasional glance and warm smile, we kept to ourselves. There wasn't any card-playing or making jokes among us like we see on television shows today. It was generally quiet, but you could hear the nurses talking, and asking their patients about pain levels and symptoms. There were also sounds of the machines ticking, the ripping of packages for new needles, and the tearing of tape to cover an injection site.

Mariano helped me to extend the seat before he left me in the company of Howard, and the nurse brought me the vomit tray without my having to ask. I'd brought popsicles in a cooler to suck on during the actual chemo injection. They were supposed to help stop the mouth sores, although all they did was make me cold.

Finding a good vein was usually challenging and that day with Howard was no exception. We chatted as the nurse attempted six times. She finally connected me to my lifeline, but left me with all those taped cotton balls dressing my forearms, which would soon bear bruises.

"What a champ!"

"My veins hide during chemo." Can you blame them? Chemotherapy hardens the veins, so they become smaller.

Howard smiled at the downplay.

It was good to get some encouragement. Though I seemed brave, I couldn't believe what I was seeing. There was pain as the nurse searched for a vein, so it distracted me from my conversation with Howard. Even today, when I receive my B12 injections, and the nurse asks me if I'm alright, I let her know, "You never get used to it."

"It was great of you to come today. I'll never forget it."

My cousin, Nick, who had visited me in the hospital following my operation, dropped by regularly once I was home. He lived at least a 45-minute car ride away, but he said he liked coming into town to buy things. "You know, some of the Italian stuff."

This made me laugh. Over time, people moved to the outskirts, and European delicacies became widely available as demand grew, turning traditional Italian fare gourmet.

Nick would spend a few hours at my house. My mother made him lunch and we'd share memories. The company, even when I wasn't feeling well, made me feel loved. Visitors broke the solitude.

Not everyone in my life could help out like this. Some cannot face suffering in a loved one. Some visit, but can't converse easily.

People's attitudes to illness differ, and have to be respected.

My advice to those wondering what they should do for someone who is seriously ill... do what you can to show they are worth the small effort. And although sharing in the final moments of a life is painful, the love that results will bring peace and closure.

Have you ever thought about what you would do if your life was at stake? I hate what the operation, chemotherapy, and radiation treatments did to my body, but the alternative was imminent death. I took what was offered, even though I suffered through those treatments. Knowing that chemo and radiation have caused me other permanent damage, I am still grateful for having had the possibility of treatment. The chemo and radiation were preventative, but the protocol saved my life.

A couple of years into my recovery, I walked into a local biscotti shop, and I ran into one of the community centre nurses that cared for me regularly at my home during treatments. She used to change my bandage for the feeding tube – which wasn't easy, since the gauze would stick to my skin as a result of leakage. She also flushed my J-Tube of any blockage using a large syringe filled with water. I would jump from the pressure as the water pushed the dried-up chemical food into my intestine.

Occasionally, she would take blood tests. If I didn't feel well, she would take care of me while I was still in bed, putting a towel underneath me so she wouldn't stain my sheets. She was much younger than I. She was always considerate, and sensitive to my weakness.

When I met her during my recovery, she had a child in a stroller, and was expecting her second shortly. It was great chatting with her. I was part of the world again, and able to socialize with those that crossed my path.

Several years later, I was involved with a committee fighting a condominium project in my neighbourhood. One of our meetings was held at a real estate agent's home, about two blocks away. As my husband and I were walking out at the end of the gathering, a woman asked us where we lived. Most of the members lived near the proposed project. She politely grilled us, making sure it was the house she was thinking of.

At first I couldn't understand her persistence, but she soon added, "I used to care for a woman there. I think it was the previous owner."

I couldn't remember her at all, but I smiled. "We are the first owners of the house. That woman was me."

She was shocked. She had mentioned during the meeting that I looked familiar, but she couldn't place me. "The lady I cared for was older."

It's nice to know I haven't aged. I certainly didn't look as presentable back then. Frailer, pale and without makeup, and with a head-kerchief to cover my awkward baldness. Of course she wouldn't recognize me now with long curly hair and pink cheeks.


When people I meet learn about my cancer, I sense the discomfort. I try to console them, so they don't feel so bad. "It was a blessing in disguise," seems to be the lesson I must teach.

Certain people are shocked to hear that. But I try to live by the same standards I teach Isabella. Why not take the good from a terrible experience? Good did come of it, and I see the gifts I receive every day since my diagnosis. If I can't appreciate the miracle I've been given, then there's no hope for me.

I am very open about the symptoms and side effects I've suffered. The physical changes, the exhaustion, the constant need to eat and drink, even the scars I refuse to hide at the beach. I've accepted these things, even though I'd rather not have them.

Accepting the unpleasant side makes life bearable. Life is never perfect.

I may be more accepting now, post cancer, but I am also less tolerant of judgement or disrespect of myself or of others. And I voice my displeasure.

Some relationships have deepened due to my increased openness. I was always a sensitive individual, but I no longer hide vulnerability. I share it. Healthy relationships cannot exist if we can't love ourselves. Self-love attracts positive connections.

When your lifestyle becomes different from that of friends, some can disappear. After I married, there was a shift in some friendships. As disappointing as that was, I realized that people cross our path... some stay, others don't.

Happily, I also experienced genuine compassion from many even after my illness. Also, the compassion was offered face-to-face.

I'm old-school. I come from a time not so long ago, when having a friend meant sharing a coffee or speaking on the telephone for more than five minutes.

Today we share emojis instead of embraces. It's a problem. Bonds are not created by just sharing pictures and writing messages full of acronyms. I prefer being present – in body and mind -- with family and friends. My contacts don't need to know where I am or what I'm doing 24 hours a day. We used to call that stalking.

That being said, I was overwhelmingly surprised by the positive reaction I received to the regular memoir excerpts I posted on my blog. I did not share pictures, and my Facebook page is quite boring. My validation comes from the real world.

To our poor children, "sharing" means posting their page on yours, and "liking" means clicking a mouse. There is a desperate need for acceptance – worse than I've seen in my younger days. I want kids to put down the electronics and live life, instead of watching a screen. They might just miss out on childhood. I worry for my daughter, reading articles that anxiety levels in children are soaring. All I can do for Isabella is be there, listening, talking, laughing at her jokes, and off-setting the trend to go virtual.

I want to teach Isabella about life, enjoy my relationships, publish my story, and make every minute count. These are challenging goals. I'll only know how my daughter turns out when she's older and I can see her happy and healthy, how strong my relationships are by the quality of the memories, how successfully this memoir's message reaches a wider audience, and I could die of old age and be content with the legacy I left behind.

Embracing life means accepting death. I've articulated some requests for my funeral. Mary and Claudia were shocked when I mentioned my favourite black lace dress hanging in my closet. "If anything happens to me, I would like to be buried in it."

Tears filled Mary's eyes. "Stop thinking like that. You're going to be fine."

To me, the conversation felt life-affirming. I've become realistic enough to know I can choose what I wear to eternity.

My daughter has a good friend whose father died unexpectedly. Her friend was only nine years old at the time, and the father, 38. Our friendship with my daughter's friend and mother have strengthened since then. The fear and familiarity that my daughter could be in that situation was real.

No one thought my life would have so much turmoil. After my hysterectomy, my niece, Claudia, shared her deepest fears.

"I'm not sure how I would have handled all that you had to endure with your health. It's too much."

"When you don't have a choice, you find the strength. And you do it for your children."

"You're really tough."

My cousin, Mario, called me just before my hysterectomy to wish me well. "My God, it's always you. Spread it around a little."

I laughed.

Years later, Mario was struck by the worst kind of cancer. From going to the emergency room for leg pain, to soon being informed that cancer had generalized, he didn't even have the opportunity to fight. I was devastated. For four months, he suffered from excruciating pain in his bones.

During a visit with him, he too told me I understood what he was going through. "You've been through worse."

*I don't know about that*, I thought. My feelings about surviving, while others perish, are conflicting. When I learn someone has cancer, I want to run to them to offer comfort. How could I have helped him? I prayed every day for my dear cousin, so he could receive the best outcome, just as I had. He was too young, the youngest of six, and the son of my aunt who died from Leukemia.

There are no answers to why one person survives cancer and another dies. I may have much experience with the illness, but even I don't know how my story will end. Doesn't everyone deserve a second chance? But I realize worthiness has nothing to do with it.

One friend from Hope & Cope who suffers a recurring cancer, I learned also experienced survivor's guilt. That clarified what I was feeling and made me feel less isolated. Watching them lose their battle and comparing our outcomes is a disturbing phenomenon. We question why we survived, and whether are end is too coming soon. Why did I get to survive? I want to be able to save others or tell them what to do to get better. But there isn't anything I could do or say that will change their outcome, or mine for that matter. Is there no way out of this epidemic?

When my husband's brother, Mike, got diagnosed with cancer in 2006 at age 47, two years after my diagnosis, I was devastated. He was already in stage IV. The cancer had spread from the colon to the liver.

I was so consumed by my own illness and treatments I now have trouble remembering all the details of Mike's case. My sister-in-law, Carole, told me recently that no one wanted to operate on Mike's liver. She and Mike eventually found a surgeon to take his case, which gave them temporary hope. He had liver surgery and also chemo, which he managed well.

During one of my visits to see him in the hospital, just before his death in 2008, his skeletal, six-foot-two body was sprawled on the hospital bed that he was never to leave. He lay uncovered and wore only shorts.

Carole and his mother were also there. He was on morphine and slept most of the time. I was standing at the end of the bed when he suddenly sat up. He was cheerful, but his eyes did not seem to see me. "Am I dying, because I feel great," he declared cheerily.

I was stunned and finally blurted out, "That's good, Mike," and he lay back down and closed his eyes.

He may have known I was there, since normally he addressed Carole in French and his mother in Italian. He was comatose. Had he heard my words? Was he aware of us standing around him?

Seeing my brother-in-law on his deathbed was terribly intimidating and frightening for me. My battle with cancer had begun four years earlier, and I was still afraid for my life. He had stopped eating and drinking. Only that stick with the tiny blue sponge touched his lips now. It was his joy.

My mother-in-law sat in the chair in the corner to the right of the bed, but could barely look his way. I cannot imagine her pain. Carole bent over him, whispering words of love.

I pictured myself lying on that bed. I was skin and bones at that time, worse than Mike ever looked. I saw my own mother crying next to me and my father silent at the side. I had to leave to keep from weeping.

Amid his brother's turmoil, Mariano shared some

emotion with me. "It's like it would be one of your sisters." It felt like he needed an excuse to cry, or was trying not to.

"I know. It hurts me too." There was a trickle of pain running through my body. During his rare moment of weakness, I put my arms around him as he sat at the dining room table that night – the same table at which we had once discussed my own fate.

When Mike died two weeks later, my husband asked me to go with him to the funeral parlour, another experience that is etched in my memory. We sat in the funeral sales office trying to pick a spot in one of the mausoleums. Carole had a plot with her family north of the city, but we needed to find another place for Mike that would be close for his mother to visit. I blocked my emotions, trying to be strong for Mariano and his family during that emotional time.

The funeral director talked about cars and the funeral service. Then he led us into another room. I wasn't sure where we were going, but when I saw the caskets, I had to stop and take a few breaths. There it was: death. There was no backing away, no shielding the eyes from the bald fact of it.

I'm not sure if Mariano understood what I was feeling. His thoughts were on his brother. I gathered my energy and treated the situation like an errand. I picked out a casket that I thought suited the family and was reasonably priced. I actually picked the one I would have wanted for my own burial. And I felt his mother would like it too. It had religious figures and gold trim on each corner. Mariano wasn't sure and wanted to consult his mother. The disjunct between this practical conversation about a purchase and the confused, painful state of our hearts unnerved us both.

At Mike's funeral, I sat at the end of the row so

that Carole and her four children – three from her first marriage who spent much of their lives with Mike – could sit close to the casket. My mother-in-law and Mariano were beside me.

The room was very large and bright, not dark like other funeral homes I've been to. I kept it together for two days, but during the sitting late one evening, I started crying. I didn't want people to worry about me and felt bad for being weak. He was Mariano's brother, not mine. I had to be strong for my husband. But I had known Mike for 10 years and loved him. He was best man at our wedding, and he loved Isabella. The loss went very deep.

In the final moments, before they closed Mike's casket for good, we each took our turn to bid farewell. My mother-in-law appeared next to me. "He loved you", she whispered. That finished off any reserve I had left.

I rested my head on the casket, and cried like a child, holding Mike's hand. I could hear Mariano quietly scolding his mother after she explained why I was weeping.

I occasionally commune with Mike and ask him about death. I ask whether I should be afraid. Perhaps it's silly, but it brings me comfort.

There are so many stories and theories about the afterlife, but I'm not at all sure what happens at death. All I know is that it will happen.

In November 2015 - my 11th year of remission – my mother-in-law was diagnosed with liver cancer. There were also lesions alongside her lungs, by the esophagus, spreading through her lymph nodes. A routine mammogram had detected a small lump in her breast five years earlier, and it was controlled with chemo therapy in pill form. About two months prior to this recent hospitalization, doctors had discovered a cancerous lymph node under her arm. We had been waiting for the hospital to give us a date to remove it when this terrible news of her metastasizing liver cancer arrived.

I happened to be the only visitor in her hospital room when the diagnosis was delivered. My mother-in-law didn't seem to understand the news, so I kept my reaction at bay. I wasn't sure how much Mariano wanted his mother to know.

Once I left the hospital, the implication of the diagnosis of a stage IV cancer crashed down on me and I began to weep. I called Mariano. I wanted him to have all the details before he headed over to the hospital after work to visit her.

My mother-in-law's prognosis was not good. A third scan, the Positron Emission Tomography (P.E.T.), ordered by her oncologist, confirmed Stage IV cancer.

On the day she was receiving her results, I had an appointment with my gynecologist to receive my own from a mammogram and breast ultrasound. They confirmed a nodule in my right breast that was smaller than a centimeter. The technician requested a six-month follow-up. My gynecologist complied. I made it to my mother-in-law's appointment, but we waited a few hours to see the oncologist.

The lymph and breast surgeries for my mother-in-law were abruptly cancelled, which deeply bothered her and Mariano. Since the cancer had metastasized, the doctors felt breast surgery would no longer be of help.

My mother had an appointment that day as well to check her breasts at the same hospital as my mother-in-law. I met up with her and my sister Mary for a while. The doctor rushed my mother to radiology after he felt a lump in her breast. It turned out to be of no concern, but it gave us a scare.

In a span of a few hours, family emotions were racing. Cancer within our families seemed so widespread that I no longer doubted its likelihood.

Mariano had lost his father to cancer 20 years earlier. He lost his brother in 2008. Now his mother was the target. Mike's death had been a big blow to her, a stress perhaps partially responsible for her aggressive cancer. Mariano was losing his entire family to cancer. He had almost lost his wife as well. He does not show much emotion, but I know that it is there.

With this genetic history, I fear for my daughter and future generations of our family.

As my mother-in-law began to show signs of furthering weakness during the next two months, tenderness and irritation in my esophagus led to concerns about recurrence. Eating often brought on acute pain and vomiting. Unhooking my brassiere more frequently helped relieve some of the pressure in the lower part of the esophagus.

My mother-in-law's nurse met with me on February 22$^{nd}$, to discuss home services offered by the local CLSC, a government medical clinic. Her health was deteriorating fast, and the hospital palliative care team thought that home palliative care would be the best plan. We were offered 30 hours a week of home nursing, beginning Thursday of the following week.

After commencing her chemo treatment, it soon became apparent that the set up could not last. She was unstable on her feet and at risk of falling. Mariano could barely lift her, and I certainly did not have the strength. I felt she should return to the hospital, but she did not want this, and Mariano refused to take her against her will.

Mariano had been spending a lot of time with his mother. She now struggled to walk, eat, and even think rationally. She kept breaking her drinking glasses, so he bought plastic ones. "When I put her to bed, she let out a sigh, like she was so happy in be in bed because she was so tired."

Mariano finally agreed that I could check on her state in the coming days, but he wanted me to speak to him before calling an ambulance.

The care-giver opened the door.

As I approached her in the living room, where she was reclining on the electric chair we convinced her to buy a year earlier, she grabbed my hand. "I can't even make it to get up," she cried in Italian.

I kissed her, and noticed her throat was moving in and out, as she struggled to breathe. "I'm going to call an ambulance," I told her. "You should go to the hospital."

"But they'll want to keep me."

"You need to be checked, Ma. You're having trouble breathing, and I want to make sure you're okay." I picked up my cell and called 9-1-1.

My sister and mother were with me so they kept her company while I called for help. My father waited in the car, since climbing stairs is painful for him. We were all returning from my father's appointment about cancerous skin lesions that keep popping up, and my annual scan (which had been moved up due to a suspicious lump my G.P. had felt in my abdomen).

Once I answered a few questions, the nurse on the telephone said not to give her anything to eat or drink. She was sending an ambulance.

The caregiver and I cleared up the kitchen, and then I dismissed her. "I'll let you know if they decide to keep her. Thank you so much for your help this week." I put my mother-in-law's pill box in my purse, and waited for the ambulance.

Once the paramedics had my mother-in-law outside, I remembered I was supposed to call Mariano before calling an ambulance. But the state of his mother's health was too worrisome to waste any time. She needed a doctor, fast. Once I explained this to Mariano, he supported the decision. I think he just didn't want to make the call himself in direct defiance of her wishes.

For the next week, her condition worsened daily. Her lungs and abdomen filled with liquid, and she became less lucid. A scan showed progression of the cancer. In the early morning of March 21$^{st}$, we received a call from the hospital doctor, telling us she was not doing well. He asked permission to commence stage IV care. Mariano told him he wanted to visit with his mother before answering.

I had to visit the hospital for scan results that day, and Mariano accompanied me before the visit to his mother. The lump turned out to be nothing, but while we were with my doctor, Mariano asked him what "stage-IV care" meant.

The doctor said it was the point when doctors realize the patient is in the final stages of the disease, and they want to be sure there is no pain. So they administer morphine.

Until that moment, I don't think Mariano understood his mother was dying. Over the past months, he may have been in denial of his mother's state, despite the fact that she was eighty-seven and cancer kept coming up on her radar. No matter what their age, it's not easy for people to say goodbye to their parents.

Mariano's eyes went wet and shiny as the doctor talked about end-of-life protocol. As Mariano walked out ahead of me, he was crying. The nurse and receptionist were confused, because they knew my scan had been fine. He turned to me with red eyes and flushed face, and smiled. "They think I'm crying for you."

Later that morning, Mariano dropped me off near the hospital entrance where his mother was, and he went to park the car. When I reached her room she was not there. A nurse stood at the door, chatting with her colleague. She asked me who I was looking for.

I said my mother-in-law's name.

"Have you spoken to the family today?" she asked, in French.

"I'm her daughter-in-law." My heart is racing.

The nurse explained that they'd been trying to get a heartbeat for five minutes. She directed me to another room nearby where my mother-in-law had been taken for emergency revival.

"Ma!" I cried, as soon as I saw her lying still on the bed. I put my hand on her forehead. Her eyes were open and her lips, parted. She made no reaction. She was gone.

# Chapter 14

# The Psychological Side

*Why do psychiatrists prescribe anti-depression pills when a situational circumstance arises? To help us forget we are dying?*

T he first time I saw a psychiatrist was in early 2005, less than one year following diagnosis. Actually, it was Susy's recommendation, and a friend of hers put me in touch with a psychiatrist at the hospital through my chemo-oncologist. I didn't think I was depressed, but I felt like speaking to an outsider so I wouldn't burden my family and friends.

I needed to know where I was headed, how to deal with daily life, and how to cope with the fear of death. Over five years, paired with visits to the fourth-floor team psychologist specialized in cancer, we discussed issues relating to home life, returning to work, and how to handle stress and fatigue.

Several visits in, on a follow-up visit with the psychiatrist, she casually brought up anti-depressants. When I said I wasn't keen, she didn't push. I explained that I'd taken so much chemo, I didn't want to overwhelm my body and brain.

Medication may fix one problem, but often it creates another. I prefer breathing exercises to help alleviate headaches or stress. A small drink – literally two tiny sips – also comes in handy.

There are so many other methods of healing available. The thought of taking medication makes me feel sick again. Dealing with emotional pain straight on is the best medicine. I wanted to know what ailed me, and to learn to handle my situation. I did not want a pill to make me forget my fear of an early death. Or make me less tired. Pills in my situation would be artificial, a mask. They would not address the underlying problem.

In fall of 2009, the psychiatrist recommended Methylphenidate for fatigue (better known as Ritalin). They're usually prescribed to patients with Attention Deficit Hyperactivity Disorder or Narcolepsy. They stopped me from sleeping, so she suggested the antidepressants again, explaining that I had situational depression. The pills would make me less emotional. Side effects included concentration and memory issues. Nausea could also arise in the first weeks.

Was she kidding me? These were all symptoms I was trying to deal with from cancer treatment. At times I get the feeling I'm in a topsy turvy world.

I still don't believe that I was depressed. I was facing death. My life had fallen apart. I was in my mid-30s with a two-year-old child and I had been told I had months to live.

By the end of 2009, I agreed to the antidepressants. The psychiatrist assured me we would start with a small dosage to see how they would affect me. I would not see any changes for about six weeks, and the pills' side effects should subside by then.

Nausea was already present, although the pills did make it worse. My dizzy spells were more frequent.

Emotionally, I felt no stronger, even after the six weeks. I promised I would stick it out to see if they helped me in the coming months. Why did I put myself through this?

We had to try a couple of different anti-depressants, and eventually settled on one. I'm not sure how long I took them, but before I decided to quit, my psychiatrist transferred me to the chief psychiatrist at the hospital and a new team. She didn't feel she could help me because cancer issues were not her specialty.

My first meeting with the new psychiatrist was intimidating. I sat in a room with her, a psychologist, and another woman. Students were watching on a television screen in another room.

I was introduced to everyone. The head psychiatrist told me that I was being assigned to the psychologist in that meeting, and that she herself would follow-up with me every two months or so to see how things were going.

The office was not like the ones you see in movies. It didn't look like a living room, with soft-lit table lamps and pretty chairs or couches. There were no paintings on the walls. An old wooden desk, vinyl low-back chairs, and the barest accessories created a spartan clinical environment.

The psychiatrist asked me about my physical and emotional health, and the psychologist, who seemed very sweet, also had her crack at me. I sat stiffly through the inquisition and then spotted the camera near the ceiling on the left. I felt doubly self-conscious imagining the students watching in the other room. The meeting lasted about an hour and a half, I think.

A day or two later, the psychiatrist called to discuss her assessment. She declared that I had major depression, which surprised me. Then, unsolicited, she offered to write my insurance company that it would be detrimental to my health to return to work.

Although I appreciated the offer, I had no intentions of working until I was fully capable, regardless of what the insurance company believed. The psychiatrist's assessment was a blow to me. What does depression feel like? How could they tell I had it? I was exhausted, cried frequently, and worried about my weight. Impatience and intolerance were also running my life. Did these symptoms amount to major depression?

The diagnosis changed me. I saw life as short and was determined to reach certain goals. If I needed to do anything, it was really up to me to go after it. My energy and finances were limited, however, and other people didn't feel the same urgency, so often I felt frustrated. Until my 10-year remission anniversary in the fall of 2014, when I finally realized I was safe, I acted like I was on borrowed time. I tried to indoctrinate Isabella, and even Mariano, who is naturally laid back, with this belief that time will run out on us.

Although I liked my former psychologist, the new one was even better suited to me. I was also relieved to be out of the oncology department and in another building, because her office was next to my chemo treatment rooms. I was constantly reminded of the miserable time I had spent on that floor. I got weak in the knees and chilled as I approached her office.

I was willing to get more involved with this new therapy group, despite the long drive from my house. In the first sessions we explored what troubled me the most, where the mental blockages were, and how the strongest emotions manifested themselves.

I tried out Eye Movement Desensitization and Reprocessing ("EMDR"), a treatment for trauma patients, that helps repressed emotions to surface.

We often ended our sessions with a breathing exercise. She would put a clip on my finger, like the ones at the hospitals that measure oxygen, and connect it to her computer. It measured my heart rate.

Prior to initiating EMDR, she asked me to create a place in my mind that felt safe.

"The safe place you create will help you relax during moments of stress. It also serves as an escape after the sessions, when you may experience disturbances during sleep or otherwise."

A cliché picture of me sitting on a lounging chair on a secluded beach came to mind. It happens to be my favourite place.

By probing, she helped me create mountains in the distance, the gentle roll of the waves, the sweet-smelling, mauve wild flowers that I could almost touch, and the warmth of a light breeze on my skin. I could imagine myself lying beside the ocean in this little haven.

My psychologist tried to help me remember the diagnosis, surgery, treatments and their aftermath. As she attempted to extract the memories, I suffered terrible headaches and nightmares. Writing this memoir has similar effects sometimes.

Healing meant I had to live through things again. I've had dreams of falling to my death, bleeding uncontrollably, having a serious illness, watching as my teeth fell out, and dying. One night, I screamed out loud in my sleep, waking my husband.

In a few sessions I wept uncontrollably, ending with day-long headaches. I wanted to stop, but the psychologist insisted we continue, since my blocked emotions and memories were coming into consciousness. I tried to comply as long as I could.

When we did EMDR, the psychologist asked me to remember a moment during the illness, or some other disturbing time, and once I began describing the scene, she would have me listen to a steady beeping sound through earphones.

"Continue with that memory." After 30 seconds or so, she stopped the beeping, and asked me what I saw. Usually, my mind went blank. I had no images relating to the day of the diagnosis or the week following. The intervals she gave me were too short to dig deeply.

"I can't get inside my head," I said. "Do I have to imagine what follows?"

"Just let it be and watch what comes to mind."

I still felt blocked. I couldn't see anything aside from the room with all the furniture and the doctor announcing my diagnosis. This memory was fragmented. And my memories of the events that followed are all jumbled chronologically.

The psychologist also tried having me follow her finger movement with my eyes. Apparently, it had a similar affect to the beeping. That process only made me dizzy, so we abandoned it.

The post-cancer pregnancy and abortion were also traumas she tried to heal with the EMDR. I wept uncontrollably during these sessions, since these memories are not repressed. The loss of my children was still fresh in my mind.

The psychologist teared up during some of those discussions. Was she feeling my pain or her own? I didn't dare ask. She was sweet and empathized with my fear of death, my grief over the loss of my children, the changes in my life, and the trepidation of abandoning my daughter.

"Are you angry that you got cancer?" My psychologist inquired on several occasions.

I shook my head.

She told me it was okay to feel anger. "It's normal to ask, 'why me?'"

But honestly, I found no reason to feel angry. Sad, yes. And confused. "I feel relieved that it wasn't someone else in my circle of friends and family."

She wasn't convinced.

I shared this question with my family. They assured me that I had not expressed anger.

Sometimes people unconsciously project emotions onto others. It's a coping mechanism, like the "mindful escape" that saved me during the worst of the traumas: that feeling of leaving my body. We are not in control. We can get damaged by life, and if we don't pay attention to our words and actions, we can damage others.

I'm not glad I got cancer. But I can acknowledge the good that resulted from it. I wouldn't wish it on anyone else, and I would never want to go through it again.

I didn't choose to get cancer, but I could choose whether or not to fight it. That's one fight I pray we all choose to engage in. The rate of success is so much greater now than when my aunt had leukemia decades ago. Statistics keep improving. I had many doubts about my own survival. Despite the uncertainty, I needed to take my chances.

My psychologist also asked me to examine how I thought others perceived my recovery.

"People forget."

"What do you mean?"

"Unless there's a crisis, people tend to dismiss that part of my life."

"Because they don't see your struggles?"

"Right... And the discomfort of confronting illness and death... I don't want to forget."

People often say, "Now you can put it behind you and move on." Hah. They should try to do this. They haven't been seriously ill. They don't know what cancer does to you. "I've been given a second chance. I don't want to abuse that."

I have learned to appreciate my life and my relationships. This doesn't mean that my life and relationships are perfect. Far from it. It just means I expect more of myself and of others. I've learned a lot about humanity.

In the final meetings with the psychiatrist, I learned that my rapid digestion can cause depression. This made sense. The constant gastric distress is a difficult part of life after cancer.

A few times, these doctors asked me whether I thought about suicide. That raised a few hackles – and my own questions. I fear dying young, so suicide wasn't an issue, even during the overwhelming sadness and exhaustion after surgery.

I'm not sure how much the EMDR treatment helped, but I certainly credit the psychologist for her sensitivity, comprehension, and helping me to heal. She gave me the human connection I needed. She helped me articulate what I was feeling and why. She assisted in bringing me to a peaceful place. She allowed me to express pain and fear.

The regular visits (as opposed to the sporadic ones I had with the first psychologist) were also helpful for healing. I was stronger than in earlier recovery years, and a bit wiser with age, so emotional recovery was now easier.

As soon as April, 2010 came around, I had decided to stop the anti-depressants. I went cold-turkey. Immediately, I noticed a big change. "It feels as though I am back from some place." I tried to describe the clarity to the psychiatrist. "I feel present in my life, aware of my surroundings... My mind is... clear." This helped me understand that the pills only clouded my judgement and masked my emotions. I should have listened to my intuition.

# Chapter 15

# They Forgot I Was Dying

*Dying for change…*

G rowing up, I was a quiet girl and writing was my sanctuary. Although I never kept a diary, writing about people and situations was my way of enjoying my simple life. I certainly had experiences I could write about, but I was never courageous enough to put my personal stories on paper.

Why would someone want to know about my life? In a large pot of broth, one tiny piece of carrot won't flavour the soup. There are bigger stories out there to attract big audiences. But I now want to tell this story about cancer. And I think people, including the patients I mentor and their families and friends, might learn something from it.

In my early writing days, research was done at the library. Today, I just do a split screen on my computer and research as I write. I have online dictionaries and a thesaurus, and find facts and statistics at the touch of a keyboard. Even grammar checks are at my fingertips.

In junior high school, when we were asked to write a journal entry for the beginning of every English class, I wrote a short story. The teacher was so impressed, he read it aloud to the class. He told me I was great with dialogue.

Perhaps writing was an access route to all I kept hidden. I joined the workforce immediately after high school. I wanted to go to college, but I was soon too busy and caught up in the corporate world. I loved the jobs I was fortunate to find, and eventually, I married, later than many of my friends. I did not mind being single. My thoughts were more about my purpose in life. I wanted to make sure I made a positive impact on people I cared about.

Today, I express my opinions more. I observe people more closely than I ever did. There are times I see things I don't want to see; but, I also now enjoy stronger relationships. Sometimes I wish I could let people be who they are, instead of wishing they were better or stronger or more virtuous. I'm not perfect, but I've learned that life is short, and that I have to take my courage in two hands and live fully. All people do. I tell my daughter to choose a career she loves, and to get the education she needs to practise it.

I really want to help others, but to do this, I have to know myself, all the dark, troubling corners, as well as the light ones. Cancer's been a great guide. I've learned a new respect for myself and to speak out when something troubles me. I also realize I need to develop tolerance. But I lose my cool when my teenage daughter doesn't listen, or when my husband doesn't share my priorities. At times, I miss the woman I used to be - quieter, more compliant and complacent. Mostly, I like what the last decade has made of me. I challenge the introvert that I am, but have come to realize that it's not so easy to change.

My short-term memory is less sharp because of

the chemo. Just the other day, I drove my daughter to day camp and left the gas stove on with a two-cup espresso pot brewing. There was a terrible smell when I returned. I had also left the milk out on the counter.

A day after that, I was washing lettuce I had picked from my garden. Leaf by leaf, I ran my fingers through in case there were any insects or dirt. I chopped them into a salad spinner. I began to fill the spinner with water again to wash the lettuce. Even more silly, I turned away to watch what was on the stove. My husband came in and turned off the water just as it was about to over-flow onto the floor.

After rearranging the contents of my kitchen drawers, I can't find anything I need for cooking because I forget that I moved them.

After being in recovery a few years, and noticing what was happening was no longer temporary, I feared returning to work. I didn't want to learn I was no longer good enough. I didn't want to disappoint anyone – especially my bosses.

I'm also self-conscious about my appearance. I think I look too skinny. I wasn't big before, but there was meat on my bones. I had some curves.

High school friends I run into say I haven't changed, which is heartening. Let's not exaggerate though. My face shows plenty of age lines. And the skin there and on my belly sags because of the weight loss.

If my cheeks and breasts could be rounder, I'd be happy. And of course there are the scars on my torso. But perhaps all people have complaints about their appear-ance in this appearance-obsessed age, not just those who have gone through cancer.

The scars are an important reminder to me to live life well, with kindness, to see beauty in ugliness, and share my feelings and insights. Cancer has brought some interesting wisdom. While I know that I'm loved, I also know the world will keep spinning when I leave it.

Following my gastrectomy, I've had important nutrient deficiencies due to malabsorption. Bone loss, vitamin B12, iron, and health of the teeth have been issues for years now. I hope there isn't anything I missed or that will come up later. My endocrinologist and other doctors are helping me with all this. I appreciate they are looking after my health and not relying solely on age-related illnesses.

At the same time, I've been told there is nothing there, but I have pain. I can eat what I want, but there are consequences. Continue to live normally, but I have limitations. "No one has ever experienced that." Maybe they haven't told you. We must be ready to look at the particulars of each case. It's time to close that book, and learn.

It's time for my annual CT-Scan, but I haven't received my appointment letter. Any time I have a medical test, anxiety rears. It's reflexive now, a deeply ingrained response. Also, any ache or pain arouses fear.

Often, I feel pain in the area I was operated and elsewhere in the torso. For several months I have been getting stabs in the lower left side of my pelvis. One day as I was driving, it started, and went on sporadically for at least 20 minutes. I drove at low speed, letting out little yelps of pain.

Since the concentration of my intestines now lay on the left side of my torso, I wonder whether the pain on that side is digestion related. The truth is, this body is a bit of a mystery. Often the doctors can't say what is going on.

After all my experience with cancer, I learned to listen to my body. This diminishes the paranoia of recurrence. I wouldn't want to ignore a health issue, and discover it is too late to do anything about it.

In speaking with patients I mentor, they often express the same anxiety relating to testing and awaiting results, and also to aches and pains. These are understandable, learned fears. They are part of survival.

About nine or 10 years into remission, my sister Mary accompanied me for scan and gastroscopy results because I was worried again about my cancer returning following unusual esophageal pain.

After about an hour's wait, my name on the intercom led us to room 15. There I waited again while the surgeon circulated the other two patient rooms.

This was the moment that everything could change. I realized that only a short time prior to testing did my fear of recurrence subside. It seems I'm never free of it. And for me, results are but for a moment that has passed, and, despite the relief, today a malignancy can be growing. I have earned the right to be cautious.

As I enter the room that day, the computer screen is facing me, open to lung X-Ray pictures. I was tempted to look at them since I had just taken one for my doctor to analyze. There was a large spot on the left side, at least one inch long by three-quarter inches wide. Familiar panic rose in my belly. My heart was racing. I felt weak at the knees. I tried not to react in front of Mary, but I was in shock. For some reason, my eyes went to the top left side of the screen, I noticed someone else's name. I was relieved, but sad for the person before me. My tests were clean.

As 2017 comes to a close, I realize I have been thinking more about life than death. I've also spent time planning for the future. Finalizing my will is on the back-burner again, although I know it must be done.

I may be entering a new phase.

# Chapter 16

# Reflections of Others

*Not all the important people in my life have contributed their thoughts here. Some preferred to keep their emotions private, and others could not put into words their feelings about the period when I was ill. But here is a sampling of perspectives on that time. My gratitude to all those who contributed to this memoir.*

*A letter from Claudia Amato:*
    *I don't think I had ever known true heartache and pain as I did when I saw my aunt, a once vibrant and strong woman, reduced to a 90-pound 'puke factory,' complete with feeding tubes and a balding head. Even then, not for one minute, did I think death could be an outcome. Call it hope, blind faith, or sheer optimism – or maybe I had never seen how terrible and cruel the world could be.*

    *In those moments where I saw how much pain she was in and how she was a whisper of who she used to be – I thought I felt real pain. Little did I know that the true pain would come years later, sitting in bed around two in the morning, nursing my third child (then just a newborn), reading this very memoir. Putting myself in her position, a mother to a two-year-old child, a wife, a daughter, a sister… Something I could not have understood at twenty years of age, it also made me realize how terrifying it must have all been. Knowing that I only ever saw her cry one time throughout the whole ordeal – "to spare US from any further pain," it was then that I understood how close I came to losing my friend, my aunt, my hero. I could not be more thankful for what she taught me, the time we have spent together, the countless conversations on my drive to work – periodically interrupted by my own bouts of morning sickness and vomiting – full circle!*

**Claudia:** You are very special to me. As the oldest grandchild (the child of my oldest sister), with only 15 years separating us in age, I love how close we've been. I love that you're happy in your life. May God bless you, Frank, and your three beautiful children. I am grateful to be here to be their Great Aunt. Thank you for pressing me to be more open about what ails me. I appreciate the opportunity to let go some times.

Thanks also for being my sounding board as I wrote this memoir. Your insights were valuable. Although feedback from outsiders was appreciated, having someone close to my story appreciate my words, makes this journey more rewarding.

Perhaps your inability to imagine my death was for the best. At age 20, I didn't want you to have to suffer. It was hard for me to see my family hurt by this illness. If I could have stopped that, I would have. But I have learned that acceptance is all we can offer, and it's the surest path to happiness. I love you, Zia Patricia.

### *A letter from Nick Varacalli:*
*"Patricia… it will be a pleasure to participate in your memoir.*

*I do remember you believing in God... the Bible clearly states that there is hope for ones that have sicknesses, or other problems, even a hope for the loved ones that passed away. It can be soothing to know that, but of course the loss or the thought of losing someone is one of the most terrible things. Human beings were not made to have those feelings. We all know that no one is content when someone close to us is sick.*

*I am not a man of many words, but I remember when my mother called me to tell me your diagnosis, those feelings of you not being there, even though we don't see each other, really affected me that day. I remember getting the call, hanging up after she told me, and afterward crying like a baby.*

*When I came to see you at the hospital, and saw your dad, he started crying, and of course once again, so did I.*

*By the way, when you write this memoir I realize that people will see that Nick Varacalli cries. I will be able to live with that............ha. I think of you often...*

*Love Nick."*

**Nick:** Your words are beautiful. I can tell you wrote from your heart. The honesty is touching, yet painful. I understand how cancer frightened everyone in my life. I'm so sorry for that. It probably hit you hard since we are the same age. It was important for me to have you write something for my memoir. I have so few memories of that time, but I remember you were often there. You made time to visit, and not out of obligation. I talk often about what you did for me. I will never forget it. God bless you. Love, Patricia, your cousin.

### A letter from Howard Greenspoon:
*"I am currently 55 years old, and there are few people of my age who have not been affected by cancer in*

*one form or another. Countless people in my circle have been directly afflicted with the disease itself, and practically everyone else can easily trace relatives who were diagnosed with some variation of this group of diseases.*

*When Patricia was first diagnosed, I recall my initial reaction of being in partial denial. How could this be? How could someone who appears to be so healthy be suffering from such a serious life-threatening disease? As the reality set in with further facts and information, I very soon realized the grim implications for Patricia and her very young family at the time.*

*In as much as our law firm's office environment had depended on Patricia's knowledge and broad contributions, I recall that work quickly became of much less importance to me. The word 'cancer' was indeed a game changer in many respects. I was far more than Patricia's employer; the two of us went back years together, and we shared intimate details of our respective lives. Patricia gained my trust, loyalty and friendship, both in our professional and personal relationship. Never would I forget the day when we were both employed at the same Montreal law firm and I informed her of my decision to leave that firm to embark upon my own quest to hang my own shingle ("Greenspoon & Associates" was born). Without hesitation, and despite the fact that I was just a fledgling attorney without more than a couple of potential clients in mind, she offered her secretarial services to me. "Pay me whatever you can afford to pay" were her words which will be forever etched in my memory.*

*We never really looked back on that decision to leave our former positions, and Patricia was instrumental in the rise of a new firm, which currently employs over 20 people on a full-time basis. From the beginning of this journey, Patricia was much more than a legal secretary. She became the bookkeeper, office manager, party plan-*

*ner, human resource point person, and generally, my faithful and dedicated 'right hand' woman who cared as much or more about the firm's success than I did.*

*All of this didn't seem to be relevant when the diagnosis came. Nothing really mattered other than whether Patricia would survive, and I became worried sick when it became clear that she was actually scheduled for immediate treatment. Her life was in danger...she had a daughter who was barely a toddler. And the prospects for full recovery were so dire that it became difficult to remain positive and hopeful.*

*I recall waiting on news after each step of the treatment; a feeling of being helpless as there was so little which I could do to help other than offering words of support and encouragement. The day that I visited Patricia during one of her chemo-therapy sessions will for always stand out in my mind. I watched as nurses were repeatedly pricking her bruised arms in search of a good vein to accept the toxic fluid that would target and eradicate the cancer. Trying to focus on Patricia and perhaps distract her from what was surely a painful ordeal, I couldn't help but notice the courage and calmness that she unexpectedly exuded throughout the session. Already, Patricia was a changed woman. What would make most people cringe, was little more than a routine event in her life; she had become a cancer patient, but with remarkable strength of character and bravery.*

*The news of her successful surgery was the first time that I remember feeling somewhat positive in regards to Patricia's prospects for a successful recovery. It was met with caution, as the normal delays would have to lapse before any real victory could be declared. A bit anticlimactic in the sense that the ultimate sense of relief would only occur five years later.*

*Patricia was not the first person close to me who*

*had been stricken with cancer, but her case particularly affected me because of her age and the special place in my heart that she had captured over the years. She hasn't come back to work since the first diagnosis, but I will for always think of her each time I revisit the inception of our firm back more than 20 years ago."*

**Howard:** Thank you for your most kind words. Your visit during my chemotherapy has been engraved in my heart too. You have been a great inspiration throughout our professional and personal years together.

You are right about feeling like partners. Your continued friendship is so important to me, and I hope always to be in your life in some capacity. An aside: I don't remember telling you "pay me whatever...!" lol... I do remember when you confided you were going on your own, and I offered you help in setting up. I had recently resigned from my post at our mutual employer, and hadn't begun searching for a new job. And the rest is history! No regrets. Love, your friend and partner, Patricia.

### *A letter from Annette Ciampanelli:*
*"To my dearest Patricia!*

*I can't recall the date or time when I was told about your condition, but I can definitely recall my emotions and all the thoughts going through my head... it was certainly a rollercoaster ride and a sad time for me - no doubt, especially for your loved ones. I remember you having your appointments and going for tests.*

*Then you were scheduled for your operation. I said a few prayers. When I visited you at the hospital, I saw the look in your eyes, and also Mariano's, that life can pass us by with a blink of an eye.*

*I not only experienced sadness, but I am so happy that I can share some time and conversation with you now that you are alive. I have known you for more than twenty years. You are a woman with great strengths, kindness, caring, and the utmost generosity that I've known in my lifetime. I consider you ultimately a true friend, and, without a doubt, having another twenty years and more of this amazing bond...*

*... Your experience is somewhat of a miracle, and it was caught in time... You are here with us enjoying day to day life experiences, and to cherish them with your loved ones. Patricia... it wasn't your time to leave us.*

*FRIENDS FOREVER!!!*
*LOVE YOU... Annette xoxoxoxox"*

**Annette:** Our relationship has deepened in recent years. Thank you for your friendship. Thank you for your sweet words.

I remember when we first met. Our desks were close, although we didn't work for the same lawyer. You and I bonded instantly, and have created even better memories since then. Other members of our group have come and gone, but you remained in my life – and for good reason. We complement each other.

Life has changed and much has happened around us since late 1989. Even after I left that firm to work with Howard, I did not want our friendship to wane. Thanks for holding on. I love you, Patricia.

*A letter from Lina Rocca:*
*"To my dear friend, Patricia:*
*Learning about your cancer left me confused, overwhelmed, and scared. The shocking news was beyond belief and devastating. I kept saying to myself that maybe there was a mistake somewhere and that the doctors would come back with something positive. It just wasn't possible. I didn't know how to react, but wanted to*

*choose the right things to say. I thought of you so often, and tried to offer you encouragement and support through your difficult time. But I will say that as time went by, I saw how strong you were, and I knew you would fight and get through all of it because you are such a strong woman, and you have a family who needs you to be there for them.*

*Having being diagnosed myself with breast cancer in 2010, left me confused, angry, and so scared. I felt depressed. All I thought about was death. I couldn't really deal with it at first – obviously in denial. I found myself overwhelmed with emotions and unable to carry out certain functions. It was a traumatic event in my life that began at the moment of the diagnosis and continued through my treatment. I kept thinking the worst, and nothing else really mattered to me. I often thought about you, and understood then the real emotional trauma you went through! I tried to stay positive as the months and years went by, which I believed was an important component for survival. My daughter was the biggest supporter and she remained so determined. She was always there for me. I realized you don't have the choice but to be strong... and that makes you stronger.*

*My cancer experience has changed a lot of things in my life. It affected my emotions and my way of thinking, and life in general. It was one of my toughest challenges. It made me realize the importance of enjoying the little things. Today I am a survivor!!*

*Patricia, you are one of the strongest women I have met. You have known suffering, pain, and struggle. But with your courage, your belief, and your determination, you fought and won the biggest battle of your life. You are a pillar of strength, and have become an inspiration to your friends and family. Today you have an appreciation and understanding of what life is all about. I am so lucky to know you and have you as a friend.*

*Love always......your friend, Lina."*

**Thank you, Lina:**

Thank you for your honesty about how my experience affected your life and your struggle. That's a gift to me, for I hope my story will inspire others. We are connected, even if the cancer we suffered is different. We all share a fear of death, isolation, and a deep hope for survival. We are also united in this fight. If somehow my struggle gave you courage, I am grateful to have been able to offer at least that. I am here when you find yourself struggling with the question, "Will I make it?"

Be well, Patricia


*A letter from Lorraine Laniel:*

*Patricia and I met in 2006 when our daughters attended a ballet school for toddlers in our neighbourhood; at a time where, little did I know, Patricia had just won the fight of her life. Over the years, we have become great friends. Nevertheless, I have always had mixed emotions about the timing of our friendship. Every one of her cancer stories makes me cry. Every one of her excerpts from the book moves me. Every "when I had cancer" comment makes me sad. I think of all her struggles and wish with all my heart that I could have been there for her because she is my dear friend; yet, I think of all her struggles and appreciate that I didn't have to see her suffer because she is my dear friend. Thank you, Lord, for your miracle.*

**Lorraine:** Hearing the perspective from someone who didn't know me during my illness is fascinating. I've been told from a few people that they would have never known, if I hadn't mentioned it. I get that, but it doesn't change the fact that I am a different person today because of what I went through battling this illness. I know that it has also allowed me to enter and build valued new friend-ships.

Thank you, Lorraine, for being in my life, and caring so much about me. It shows, and I appreciate your every effort to help me out of my shell.

# Chapter 17

# The Return

*Every day is a miracle for me. I thank God
for this second chance.*

We know that death will come, we just don't
know when. At 35, I was not ready. I have
certainly changed over the last 13 years, but the change
isn't due to cancer alone. It comes from receiving the
chance to live, to build better relationships, to be a better
role model, and offer inspiration to those that need it.

And after all these years, I'm still in recovery,
physically and emotionally. I will be for life. Volunteering has taught me that just as one person dies of cancer,
another begins his fight. Paying attention to the unending
cycle of death and life keeps me humble and available to
others.

Amidst all the suffering, there can be happiness.
Life is not a fairy tale, but if we can find a few moments
each day to savour the peace and love, the fear of death
diminishes. It took me many years, but I am finally able
to see all that I deserve in this life.

This journey is for Isabella's sake. If I am not

happy, I know that her chances of being happy are much lower. I am confident that I have shown her how a human being can be strong in difficult times. Hopefully, she will never have to prove what a clever student she is, but life has a habit of testing us. Hopefully I will be around to help her through those tests, and give her all my love and support. If I am not, I implore her to use the tools I've given her to surpass any grievance along her way to meet me.

I've dropped a lot of fear since my diagnosis. And I've come to know myself better. Embracing life has taught me to let people get closer to me. I trust enough to seek help when I need it. I'm not afraid to show my imperfect life, instead of hiding my problems away.

Perhaps now, instead of seeing myself in the casket at funerals, I can see my resolve to lead a happy, balanced life. I've made peace with the dead and the dying. Time has given me that freedom. Talking with others has allowed me to feel safe enough to look ahead and plan for the future. This faith doesn't arrive overnight. It took patience to learn acceptance and self-love.

For many years I thought about death and the recurrence of cancer. But thinking about it did not bring peace. My attitude was still tense and fearful. If you don't take a treatment to cure a disease, it will worsen, and perhaps even kill you. If you don't take the necessary measures to heal your traumatized mind, you might destroy yourself and others around you.

Therapy, friends and family, prayer, and this memoir have been helpful measures. I have emerged a stronger and healthier woman from this experience, with so much more to offer. I have finally broken free from fear of cancer. It is alright to live my life as it has evolved, without guilt, without the need to justify the changes. I can be me – whoever that may be. I am happy living each day and discovering myself anew.

I'll probably have to live the rest of my life wondering if people are judging my second navel, and listening to family members introduce me as "the one that was sick" instead of "the youngest of the four daughters." I will definitely live with worry about recurrence for the rest of my days. But these preoccupations are no longer strong or crippling. I can live with the chronic fatigue, the consequences of my surgery and treatments, and not being able to do much on my own. I also weigh myself much less often.

I was born of my mother and am privileged to have experienced the birth of my own child. I've completed the circle of life. My mother supported me when I was ill, and when my daughter needs me, I can be there. Isabella's birth gave me a purpose and love that cannot be broken.

This memoir was written especially for those who suffer from life-threatening illnesses. If this description includes you, my only wish is that you find words here that inspire you. I beat odds and statistics. May this story help you on your own journey, and may you heal that part of you that prevents you from feeling peace, whatever your medical outcome.

I don't hold myself in high esteem today because I have beaten fear. I merely accepted the consequences of stomach cancer.

A recent research on the site of the *Canadian Cancer Society's Stomach Cancer* page, I learned (or probably forgot that I had read it previously) that having blood type A is also a risk for stomach cancer. Although the reason is unknown, I had to double check what my type was. And indeed I am blood type A.

# Chapter 18

# How to Fight Cancer

H ere are a few tools to help you through some difficult times:

1. Beat it with a stick. There will be a struggle. But overcome it or not, you are a hero.

2. Give yourself a reason to fight. If you
don't have one (and we all have at least one – a
child, partner, friend, pet, getting up in the morning
to see the sunshine, being too young, just because…), I will provide one… fight for yourself,
because you deserve a great life.

3. Even if you are not religious, find something that inspires you. You can derive strength
throughout your battle with cancer if you know
what is important to you. I found peace and trust
that God knows my destiny.

4. Don't give up. Even through horrific
treatment symptoms, I completed the protocol.
Look at the chance that it gave me.

5. Get professional help – it is so important
to understand you are not alone in your fight. I did-
n't want to burden my family and friends with my
fears. My psychologist made me feel it was alright
to cry when I needed to.

6. Don't be angry with the world. Find peace
through prayer, meditation, support… Whatever

time you have left should not be wasted on anger. Pushing away those that love you won't change your diagnosis or affect the outcome. Cancer isn't their fault (or yours).

7. Discover your coping mechanism. Think about how you have handled other traumatic situations. Search for something you love to do so it distracts you. Talk about what you're going through, don't suffer in silence. What is your state of mind, and how can it help you cope? Weird though it was, separating from my body periodically throughout my ordeal helped me get through.

8. Give back, if you've been given another chance. Find happiness and fulfillment in helping others. Your help is desperately needed, and for you, I guarantee it will be powerful medicine.

9. Search hard for an appropriate medical institution and team. That was the main priority after diagnosis.

10. Share your love with those closest to you. This may be tough if you are unpractised. Remember that just being with someone or holding their hand lets them know they are important. This goes for all of us.

Nothing you do will ensure survival. Cancer is not easy and the treatments can be just as bad. Facing death is traumatizing, no matter how balanced you are. But attitude really helps. And these top 10 are good reminders.

Life is, essentially, out of our control. We must do our best to accept what comes our way, and take proper steps to fight, or eventually submit to our destiny. I cannot imagine myself leaving this world angry, after the opportunity I've been given. There have been bad, ugly times, for sure. But there is a lot to give thanks for: the beautiful family that surrounds me, the husband who has stood by me, and especially my beautiful daughter, Isabella. And then there are the friends who have crossed my path and inspired me in this life.

I want to be healthy. I want to be happy. I want to write. Of course, I'd love to have success in my writing career, now that I've set out to do it publicly. But that is icing on my mother's four-layer cake.

# About the Author

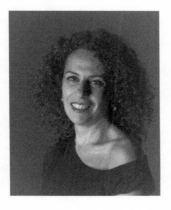

Faced with a life-threatening illness, Patricia Rodi's life as a first-time mother, corporate paralegal, and office manager comes to a halt. Recovery takes her back to writing, and 17 years following her diagnosis, she publishes her memoir about her incredible journey. She is a member of the Quebec Writers' Federation, and lives in Montreal, Canada with her husband and daughter.

**You can reach PATRICIA RODI at the sites below:**

 https://LivingAfterCancerBlog.Wordpress.com

**PODCAST**
https://Anchor.fm/patricia-rodi
(or wherever you get your podcasts)

 https://www.linkedin.com/in/patricia-rodi-45b659218

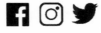

@PatriciaRodiMtl

Manufactured by Amazon.ca
Bolton, ON

24519090R00122